Chemotherapy and Pharmacology for Leukemia in Pregnancy

Carolina Witchmichen Penteado Schmidt
Kaléu Mormino Otoni

Editors

Chemotherapy and Pharmacology for Leukemia in Pregnancy

Guidelines and Strategies for Best Practices

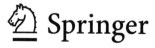 Springer

Editors
Carolina Witchmichen Penteado Schmidt
Pediatric Oncology Pharmacist
& Scientific Writer
Curitiba
Paraná
Brazil

Kaléu Mormino Otoni
Pronutrir Nutritional Support
and Chemotherapy Ltda
Fortaleza
Ceará
Brazil

ISBN 978-3-030-54057-9   ISBN 978-3-030-54058-6   (eBook)
https://doi.org/10.1007/978-3-030-54058-6

This Springer imprint is published by the registered company Springer Nature Switzerland AG
The registered company address is: Gewerbestrasse 11, 6330 Cham, Switzerland

Preface

One of our great challenges as health professionals in hematology is that we already work with a particular group of patients that requires specialized knowledge. This group of hematological patients is already individualized among the various hematological diseases. Even when we identify the type of leukemia in patients, their genetic conditions, and the risk group they belong to, they can yet be part of an even more restricted group: that of pregnant patients.

Professionals who work with leukemia diagnosis and treatment race against time, and when a patient requires greater care, the lack of widely defined and well-standardized protocols makes the work of these professionals difficult, and it reflects in the health of both patients: mother and fetus. As there is little data on the treatment of leukemia during pregnancy, Kaléu and I decided to edit this book to save time for professionals involved in the care of pregnant women with leukemia. We gather a great team that includes pharmacists in pediatrics, oncology, hematology, clinical pharmacy, and pharmacovigilance; physicians in hematology, obstetrics, gynecology, infectious diseases, and palliative care; in addition to researchers. Our team of specialists gathered and curated the available information in addition to making it as transparent and practical as possible for daily use.

Carolina Witchmichen Penteado Schmidt
Pediatric Oncology Pharmacist and Scientific Writer
Author of the Springer books: *Hematopoietic Stem Cell Transplantation for Pharmacists: The Gold Standard to Practice*; *Pediatric Oncologic Pharmacy: A Complete Guide to Practice*; *Chemotherapy in Neonates and Infants: Pharmacological Oncology for Children Under 1 Year Old*; and *Drug Therapy and Interactions in Pediatric Oncology: A Pocket Guide*. Author of various children's books about cancer, including the award-winning *Chubby's Tale: The true story of a teddy bear who beat cancer* and the best-selling book *Bald is Beautiful: A letter for a fabulous girl*.

Kaléu Mormino Otoni

Oncology Pharmacist and Professor, ProNutrir Nutritional Support and Chemotherapy. Specialist in Oncological Hospital Pharmacy. MBA in Health Management.

Curitiba, Paraná, Brazil   Carolina Witchmichen Penteado Schmidt
Fortaleza, Ceará, Brazil   Kaléu Mormino Otoni

Contents

Contributors

Gustavo Alves ISTAART – The Alzheimer's Association International Society to Advance Alzheimer's Research and Treatment, Chicago, IL, USA

ASHP – American Society of Health-System Pharmacists, Bethesda, MD, USA

Department of Pharmacy, SENAC University Center, São Paulo, Brazil

Karla Rodrigues Andrade Oncological Pharmaceutical Care Center at Hospital Sírio-Libanês, São Paulo, Brazil

Maria Cecília Borges Bittencourt Centro Paulista de Oncologia and Hospital 9 de Julho, São Paulo, Brazil

Ana Costa Cordeiro Centro Paulista de Oncologia and Hospital 9 de Julho, São Paulo, Brazil

Pedro Mikael da Silva Costa Laboratory of Experimental Oncology, Research and Development of Medicines Center, Universidade Federal do Ceará, Fortaleza, Brazil

Giancarlo Fatobene Hospital das Clínicas, University of São Paulo and Hospital Sírio-Libanês, São Paulo, Brazil

Rossana Pulcineli Vieira Francisco Hospital das Clínicas, University of São Paulo, São Paulo, Brazil

Celina de Jesus Guimarães Laboratory of Experimental Oncology, Research and Development of Medicines Center, Universidade Federal do Ceará, Fortaleza, Brazil

Fundação Centro de Controle de Oncologia do Estado do Amazonas, Manaus, Brazil

Ana Maria Kondo Igai Hospital das Clínicas, University of São Paulo, São Paulo, Brazil

Andrea Maria Novaes Machado Stem Cell Transplantation Team of the Hospital Israelita Albert Einstein, São Paulo, Brazil

ABC Medical School, Santo André, Brazil

Aline Rebeca de Sousa Magalhães Catholic University Center of Quixadá, Quixadá, Ceará, Brazil

Sarah Sant' Anna Maranhão Laboratory of Experimental Oncology, Research and Development of Medicines Center, Universidade Federal do Ceará, Fortaleza, Brazil

Rafael Fernandes Pessoa Mendes Hospital Sírio-Libanês, São Paulo, Brazil

Karla Bruna Nogueira Torres Mormino Catholic University Center of Quixadá, Quixadá, Ceará, Brazil

Gilmar de Souza Osmundo Junior Hospital das Clínicas, University of São Paulo, São Paulo, Brazil

Kaléu Mormino Otoni Pronutrir Nutritional Support and Chemotherapy Ltda, Fortaleza, Ceará, Brazil

Claudia Pessoa Laboratory of Experimental Oncology, Research and Development of Medicines Center, Universidade Federal do Ceará, Fortaleza, Brazil

Danilo Belchior Ponciano Bone Marrow Transplant Units of Hospital Sírio Libanês, São Paulo, Brazil

Bruno Azevedo Randi Hospital 9 de Julho, São Paulo, Brazil

William Rotea Jr. Oncology Pharmacist, São Paulo, Brazil

Ranieri Sales de Souza Santos Catholic University Center of Quixadá, Quixadá, Ceará, Brazil

Mariângela Borges Ribeiro da Silva Uiversidade Federal do Paraná (UFPR), Curitiba, Brazil

Vinicius Ponzio da Silva Hospital 9 de Julho, São Paulo, Brazil

Carolina Witchmichen Penteado Schmidt Pediatric Oncology Pharmacist & Scientific Writer, Curitiba, Paraná, Brazil

Polianna Mara Rodrigues de Souza Stem Cell Transplantation Team of the Hospital Israelita Albert Einstein, São Paulo, Brazil

Oxford International Center for Palliative Care, Oxford, UK

Pain Committee for the Elderly of the Brazilian Society for the Study of Pain-SBED, São Paulo, Brazil

Bioethics Committee of Hospital Israelita Albert Einstein, São Paulo, Brazil

Oncology and Hematology Center of Hospital Israelita Albert Einstein, São Paulo, Brazil

Chapter 1
Introduction

Gustavo Alves

1.1 Introduction

Statistics on the frequency of malignant diseases in pregnant women points to 1 in 1000 cases. The incidence of leukemia in pregnant women can vary from 1 in 75,000 to 1 in 100,000 cases, and acute leukemia represents the majority of leukemia cases during pregnancy. Immediate treatment is essential for acute leukemia cases, even with the risks involving pregnancy; if not treated immediately, the risk of maternal mortality is increased [5]. In summary, avoiding the risks of chemotherapy in the first trimester and postponing postpartum treatment is not a preferable strategy [1–4].

From the physiological point of view, a pregnant woman's body naturally undergoes changes during pregnancy, which makes the diagnosis of leukemia even more difficult. There is a great risk that this diagnosis may be delayed or even neglected for some time, as some common symptoms of pregnancy may be mistaken for symptoms of leukemia. We can highlight fatigue, shortness of breath, and weakness in general as the most important symptoms. In addition, anemia and leukocytosis may be present in pregnancy at the same time as they are considered common findings in leukemia [6]. All the time lost in effective diagnosis can cause a great loss in the treatment and quality of life of the patient.

As previously stated, the diagnosis of leukemia is not simple, requiring morphological, immunophenotypic, and cytogenetic evaluations of bone marrow samples. A bone marrow biopsy is performed safely under local anesthesia only in pregnant

G. Alves (✉)
ISTAART – The Alzheimer's Association International Society to Advance Alzheimer's Research and Treatment, Chicago, IL, USA

ASHP – American Society of Health-System Pharmacists, Bethesda, MD, USA

Department of Pharmacy, SENAC University Center, São Paulo, Brazil

© Springer Nature Switzerland AG 2021
C. W. P. Schmidt, K. M. Otoni (eds.), *Chemotherapy and Pharmacology for Leukemia in Pregnancy*, https://doi.org/10.1007/978-3-030-54058-6_1

1

women, a simple procedure performed without causing any harm to the fetus, obviously being careful not to pose a risk of infection [6].

1.2 Ethical Dilemmas

Many ethical dilemmas can be observed in issues related to the treatment of any disease in a pregnant woman, starting with the safety of the drugs used, since in most cases, teratogenic events are only recognized and evaluated after the occurrence of damage caused. In general, some choices must be made, always aiming at the preservation of human dignity and considering the presence of one or more fetuses. Using a drug with potent antitumor action on a pregnant woman will trigger unmanaged and managed consequences.

1.3 Multidisciplinary Team

The Leukemia during pregnancy is in itself a medical emergency, due to its progression and rapid progress, and requires redoubled attention. The work of the multidisciplinary team is important because in addition to neonatologists and pediatricians, it will gather oncologists, hematologists, social workers, psychologists, and pharmacists, among others. Since diagnosis to treatment, the patient plays a fundamental role in deciding [7] whether to adopt a more conservative therapy or risk all the more for therapeutic success.

1.4 Statistics and Concept

1.4.1 United States of America

In the United States, monitoring of disease-related indices and other health impact indices are very effective, often serving as a basis for epidemiological studies and assessments, even to other countries. Regarding the number of new cases and mortality rates per 100,000, the following numbers were calculated:

The number of new cases of leukemia was 14.1 per 100,000 men and women per year. The rate of deaths was 6.5 per 100,000 men and women per year. These rates are age-adjusted and based on 2012–2016 cases and deaths. Approximately 1.6% of men and women will be diagnosed with leukemia at some point during their lifetime, based on 2014–2016 data. Prevalence of Leukemia: In 2016, there were an estimated 414,773 people living with leukemia in the United States [8].

In Brazil (INCA 2018) [9]:

- Estimates of new cases: 10,800
- 5940 men
- 4860 women
- Number of deaths: 6837
- 3692 men
- 3145 women

Leukemia is a disease of unknown origin with white blood cells of malignant character. Its main feature is the accumulation of leukemic cells in the bone marrow, replacing normal cells. In the bone marrow, cells are produced, giving rise to white and red blood cells. In patients with leukemia, these blood cells that have not yet matured will mutate into cancer cells. There is then a process of gradual replacement of normal cells with cancer cells [9].

In a pregnant woman, the damage caused by leukemia, regardless of type, is enormous, even greater than in an adult individual. This process occurs because homeostasis, common in pregnant women, is a balance point for metabolism, energy expenditure and cell multiplication. Any damage in this physiological condition brings exponential damage that may also extend to the fetus.

1.4.2 Risk Factors for Leukemia

It is not possible to clearly and accurately determine all risk factors as well as causes for leukemia; however, it is known, that benzene and ionizing radiation are determining environmental factors for acute leukemia. Although without defined causes, the association of some elements may increase the risk of developing some specific types of leukemia [9]:

- Exposure to substances used in agricultural management, such as pesticides, diesel, solvents, and dust: leukemias.
- Chemotherapy: acute myeloid leukemia and acute lymphoid leukemia.
- Smoking: acute myeloid leukemia.
- Ionizing radiation (X-rays and gamma rays) from radiotherapy: acute myeloid leukemia and acute lymphoid leukemia. The degree of risk will depend on age, radiation dose, and exposure to agents.
- Exposure to formaldehyde, which is a product used in the textile, chemical industry, and also used in hospitals, laboratories, clinics as a solvent, histological fixative, disinfectant, and antiseptic, can cause leukemia.
- Rubber production: leukemia.
- Down syndrome and other hereditary factor-related diseases: acute myeloid leukemia.
- Family history: acute myeloid leukemia and chronic lymphoid leukemia.
- Myelodysplastic syndrome and other blood disorders: acute myeloid leukemia.

- Benzene: substance widely used in the chemical industry and in the composition of fuels such as gasoline – acute and chronic myeloid leukemia and acute lymphoid leukemia.
- Age: the risk of acquiring leukemia increases with age, except for acute lymphoid leukemia, which is more common in children. All others mostly affect the elderly.

We can correlate many of the above situations with the occurrence of leukemia, manifesting in the gestational period. Many women prefer to have children later in life. Although the number of smokers worldwide has decreased, still the number of female smokers is large. And we must not forget the factors linked to occupational contamination and family inheritance (hereditary).

1.5   General Aspects of Treatment

The most commonly diagnosed cancers in pregnant women are cervix, breast, melanoma, lymphoma, and leukemia [16].

In 1856, Rudolph Virchow, considered the father of modern pathology, described the first scientific work on leukemia, precisely in a pregnant woman. He already claimed that this disease caused molecular or structural changes in cells. Since Virchow's discovery until 1995, more than 500 cases of leukemia have been reported in pregnant women [6], most of them being acute and predominantly myeloid [10].

Acute leukemia in pregnant women causes anemia, thrombocytopenia, and neutropenia; and infections may occur due to bone marrow failure caused by the malignancy of the disease [7]. The risk of increased susceptibility to infections increases with leukemia, as well as cytopenia and autoimmune phenomena. Infections are a serious maternal and fetal risk problem, and it is important to remember that not all antibiotics can be used during pregnancy. It is essential to assess the presence of herpes virus and cytomegalovirus during leukemia due to the increased risk of reactivation [11].

Cytopenias can cause infections and bleeding, which are considered very serious events during gestational period. In the spinal cord failure caused by leukemia, red blood cell and platelet transfusions are used to maintain hemoglobin levels of approximately 10 g/dL and platelet counts in the range >50–100 × 109/L (with close monitoring of platelet level) at delivery [12].

Pregnant women with acute promyelocytic leukemia (ALI) require special vigilance and care, as the most common manifestations of ALI include medical emergencies such as pancytopenia, intravascular coagulation, and hyperfibrinolysis [13]. Chemotherapy in the first trimester of pregnancy significantly increases the risk of miscarriage, fetal malformation, and fetal death [14].

As for the diagnosis of leukemia in pregnant women, it will be the same as in nonpregnant women; however, certain radiological evaluations that may affect the fetus may not be performed in pregnant women [7]. Although biopsy can be performed during pregnancy, it should be avoided; however, for accurate confirmation, techniques such as peripheral blood microscopy, flow cytometry or molecular analysis are required [10].

When the diagnosis of leukemia is made in the first trimester of pregnancy, termination of pregnancy may be considered [15, 18]. During the second and third trimesters, chemotherapy treatment will rarely cause congenital malformations, but the risk of prematurity, *fetal growth restriction*, neonatal neutropenia, and sepsis should be considered [15].

The treatment of a cancer patient during pregnancy is challenging, mainly due to the effects that can be caused to the fetus. The effects will be influenced by factors such as time and frequency of drug exposure and the ability of drugs to cross physiological barriers such as the blood-brain barrier and the placental barrier. Other issues to be evaluated include diagnosis and gestational period [17].

For ethical and moral reasons, no studies have been performed on pharmacokinetic profiles of chemotherapy drugs in pregnant women. Thus, the doses that pregnant women receive from chemotherapy are exactly the same as those of nonpregnant women. In pregnancy, the blood volume increases by up to 50%, and the same occurs with the renal clearance rate that also increases; therefore, the serum concentration of the drug can be reduced. In a pregnant woman, the hormonal and metabolic changes associated with pregnancy should be considered [15].

Chemotherapy in leukemia inhibits placental trophoblast migration and proliferation in the first trimester of pregnancy, which may partially explain the lower birth weights of newborns whose mothers received chemotherapy [19]. The trophoblast is the outer layer of the blastocyst and contributes to endometrial implantation and placental formation. It is essential to mention that chemotherapy drugs disrupt vital cell functions during some phases of the cell cycle [15, 20].

Table 1.1 describes and the consequences of chemotherapy in the treatment of leukemia during the first, second, and third trimesters of pregnancy.

At King Faisal Hospital and Research Center in Riyadh, the capital of Saudi Arabia, a research was conducted on 32 patients who developed leukemia during pregnancy, with long-term follow-up. The types of primary hematologic malignancies were CML (11 patients), acute promyelocytic leukemia (ALI) (5 patients), and non-M3 AML (8 patients). Spontaneous abortions occurred in 14 patients and therapeutic abortions in 2 patients, while 16 live births were delivered at

Table 1.1 Chemotherapy in pregnancy [21]

Leukemia (type)	First trimester of pregnancy	Second trimester of pregnancy	Third trimester of pregnancy
Acute leukemia	Abortion	Cytarabine and doxorubicin induction therapy	Induction of labor and initiation of therapy
Acute promyelocytic leukemia	Abortion	Doxorubicin and trans retinoic acid	Induction of labor and initiation of therapy
Chronic myeloid leukemia (CML)	Interferon-alpha	Interferon-alpha or imatinib	Interferon-alpha or imatinib

30–41 weeks of gestation. Regarding the results obtained from the mothers, this research found that 19 patients were dead; 7 patients lost follow-up, and only 6 patients were alive. Of the 32 patients evaluated, 19 underwent hematopoietic stem cell transplantation (HSCT) to control their primary hematologic malignancies. At long-term follow-up, 14 transplant recipients were dead and only 5 transplant patients survived. Negatively, we can conclude from this case that the long-term prognosis of pregnant women with leukemia is poor, even with HSCT in high-risk patients [22].

In another study conducted in Japan, 16 patients with leukemia during pregnancy were evaluated between 2001 and 2011. Of the 16 patients evaluated, 9 had chronic myeloid leukemia (CML), 5 had acute lymphoid leukemia (ALL), and only 2 had developed acute myeloid leukemia (AML). Almost half of CML patients received treatment with imatinib, which was discontinued in three patients after the first trimester and one after the second trimester. Of these nine CML patients, six were treated with hydroxyurea and/or interferon, while the remaining three patients had no complementary treatment following the use of imatinib. Anemia was developed in four patients and thrombocytopenia in one patient. Acute leukemia was diagnosed in seven patients: two during the first trimester, two during the second trimester of pregnancy, and three during the third trimester of pregnancy. Two ALL patients had therapeutic abortion. Four ALL patients received chemotherapy in the first trimester of pregnancy. All patients with acute leukemia had thrombocytopenia, while four patients developed febrile neutropenia. At birth, the average gestational age was 32 weeks, with two reported perinatal deaths. In this study, it was possible to conclude that fetal and maternal morbidity is high in pregnant women with acute leukemia, while in pregnant women with chronic leukemia, fetal and maternal prognosis may be more favorable and management of complications is easier compared to acute leukemia [23].

Vertical transmission of leukemia from mother to fetus is rare and uncommon, thanks to the placental barrier and the immune system of the fetus. Chemotherapeutic agents have low molecular weight, so most of them can cross the placental barrier and reach the fetus. When treating a pregnant woman with antineoplastic drugs, we should consider the physiological changes that occur in the woman's body and the potential changes in drug metabolism and excretion. Increased renal clearance and hepatic oxidation of drugs occur during pregnancy, which may negatively influence the outcome of the protocols, as well as reducing the safety of these drugs [7].

Some medicines used to treat leukemia may be harmful in pregnancy:

- Imatinib: it is a tyrosine kinase inhibitor which blocks proliferation and induces the apoptosis process. This is related to some fetal abnormalities and abortion and is shown to be teratogenic in mice. Some studies claim that it can be safely used throughout pregnancy, but studies are lacking to prove its safety in the first trimester of pregnancy [11, 24].
- Nilotinib: it is a tyrosine kinase inhibitor which blocks proliferation and induces the apoptosis process [24]. Animal studies suggest that the use of this drug in pregnancy is related to mortality, miscarriage, and reduced gestational weight at

a dose of 300 mg/kg/d. Other authors suggest that nilotinib has no teratogenic action, determining successful pregnancies in patients [24].

- Trans retinoic acid: it participates in the regulation of transcription of target genes that control cell proliferation, differentiation, and apoptosis. According to studies, this drug causes teratogenic effects, such as craniofacial alterations, neural tube defects, cardiovascular malformations, and thymic aplasia, mainly in the first trimester of pregnancy. Spontaneous abortions occur in 40% of cases. In the second and third trimesters of pregnancy, there is less risk of teratogenic effects [19, 25].
- Hydroxyurea: it inhibits DNA synthesis [26]. In rats, the use of hydroxyurea has been shown to increase the risk of teratogenic effects. Some studies report that it can cause miscarriage, intrauterine growth retardation, and congenital malformation without specifying exactly which trimester is most at risk [19, 27].
- Cytarabine: this is an antimetabolite, acting as a false substrate for reactions necessary for DNA replication and RNA synthesis. The recommendation is to avoid the use of cytarabine throughout pregnancy. During the first trimester, it can cause severe limb malformations, and its use in the second and third trimesters is related to transient cytopenias, intrauterine fetal death, intrauterine growth retardation, and neonatal death from sepsis and gastroenteritis [19, 28].
- Methotrexate: this is an antimetabolite which acts as a false substrate for reactions necessary for DNA replication and RNA synthesis. Similar to most drugs, it should also be avoided during the first trimester of pregnancy. If really needed, it can be used in the second and third trimesters of pregnancy. Studies do not specify exactly which complications may occur for the mother and the fetus [19, 28].
- Rituximab: the mechanisms of this drug are antibody-dependent cell-mediated cytotoxicity, complement-dependent cytotoxicity, and apoptosis induction [29]. It has a low risk of teratogenicity compared to other drugs but should be avoided during the first trimester of pregnancy. Some studies and research indicate that rituximab can be safely used in the second and third trimesters of pregnancy [19].
- Thalidomide and Lenalidomide: they have anti-inflammatory activity, are immunomodulatory, and inhibit anti-apoptosis effects. They trigger antiangiogenic effects and inhibit the production, release and signaling of tumor necrosis factor-α (TNF-α) and interleukin-6 (IL-6) and lead to cytotoxicity mediated by T30 cells. They may cause teratogenic effects and should be avoided during pregnancy [19].

Like drugs, some of the tests used to diagnose leukemia during pregnancy may not be safe [15]:

- Excisional biopsy and bone marrow biopsy: safe in pregnancy.
- Ultrasound: safe in pregnancy.
- Computed tomography and PET scan: may cause carcinogenic, teratogenic effects or miscarriage during pregnancy.
- Magnetic resonance imaging (MRI) and use of gadolinium: MRI can be safely used during the second and third trimesters of pregnancy only if there is a strong

reason for it, as it poses a risk to the fetus. The use of gadolinium as a contrast is dangerous because it crosses the placenta and affects the development of the fetus, producing malformations and restricting growth. The use of iodinated contrast agents is not recommended as they can cross the placenta and cause depression of thyroid function.

1.6 Postpartum Effects of Chemotherapy on Mothers with Leukemia

At the end of pregnancy, chemotherapy should not be administered as it may lead to childbirth without bone marrow recovery. Some common complications occur during childbirth; however, thrombocytopenia, characteristic of leukemia, can lead to excessive bleeding in caesarean section or normal delivery. Severe anemia can complicate delivery of oxygen to the fetus. Obstetric infections can become very serious if neutropenia is present [30]; hence, chemotherapy should be discontinued 3 weeks before delivery for fetal placental excretion of drugs, which reduces the risk of neonatal myelosuppression [15].

Planning all chemotherapy sessions is critical, so that the risks are minimized. A caesarean section may be required in a patient with leukemia, neutropenia, or thrombocytopenia. After childbirth, it is recommended that breastfeeding begin 2 weeks after the last administration of chemotherapeutic agents because of the risk of toxicity involved. Even in small concentrations, drugs can be secreted into breast milk and cause significant harm to the fetus. Following chemotherapy in a leukemia patient, it is recommended to wait between 6 months and 2–5 years to allow oocytes to recover from possible drug damage during treatment [31].

1.7 Leukemias During Pregnancy

1.7.1 Acute Myeloid Leukemia in Pregnancy

Acute Myeloid Leukemia in Pregnancy is a type of cancer of the white blood cell myeloid line, characterized by the rapid proliferation of malignant and abnormal cells, the blasts, which do not mature without performing their functions and accumulate in the bone marrow. As a result, it interferes with the production of other cells [32]. AML occurs quite frequently in young adults and the elderly. Thus, more data are available for the management of AML in pregnant women [6, 10]. AML has no aggressive malignancy, but delayed initiation of chemotherapy has adverse consequences for the mother. Therefore, careful evaluation should be performed to find a balance between the consequences of intensive chemotherapy on the fetus and mother. Also, check the consequences of postponing treatment to the mother [6, 10].

The possibility of long-term consequences of chemotherapeutic cytotoxicity on the mother's future fertility should be considered [10, 33].

There are therapeutic regimens and protocols for the treatment of AML, and these include the use of anthracyclines (daunorubicin, idarubicin, doxorubicin), antimetabolites (cytarabine), topoisomerase II inhibitors (etoposide), monoclonal antibodies (gemtuzumab), and multikinase inhibitors [10]. AML induction regimens are based on a combination of cytarabine and anthracycline, while other combinations of intensive chemotherapies are used in consolidation therapy [6, 7]. There are sufficient data on the use of cytarabine and anthracyclines during pregnancy, except in the first trimester; however, there is a lack of information on the administration of gemtuzumab and multikinase inhibitors in pregnant women with AML [6, 10]. Experience with the use of anthracyclines in pregnancy is limited to the administration of doxorubicin and daunorubicin, since idarubicin, being more lipophilic, may be related to higher rates of fetal complications [7, 33].

There are many reports of successful management of AML in pregnancy and few reports of vertical transmission of acute leukemia from mother to fetus [34, 35]. Spontaneous remission of acute leukemia after pregnancy has been reported and the following rare forms of AML have been reported: erythroleukemia, AML with granulocytic sarcoma causing spinal cord compression, and AML mimicking HELLP (hemolysis, elevated liver enzymes and low platelet counts) syndrome [36].

Although AML is a rare event during pregnancy, there is a clear risk to life for both mother and fetus. AML diagnosed during pregnancy should be treated immediately, as higher maternal mortality is associated with delayed initiation of treatment. However, the decision regarding the choice of treatment for AML in pregnancy will depend on the case. If AML is diagnosed during the first trimester of pregnancy, termination of pregnancy should be discussed and chemotherapy should be initiated [34, 35, 37–40].

Management of AML diagnosed during the second and third trimesters of pregnancy is often difficult because simply delaying the initiation of chemotherapy sessions entails significant risk for the mother, and administration of antineoplastic drugs induces fetal death, prematurity, malformations, and congenital infections [39]. Some studies state that chemotherapy may be safe during the second and third trimesters of pregnancy, and that chemotherapy with cytarabine and idarubicin in AML in the second trimester of pregnancy may be associated with fetal heart malformations. These are conflicting issues which, as a rule, run into the risk to the fetus, most likely in the first trimester of pregnancy. The choice of chemotherapy, specifically in the first trimester of pregnancy, will always be a challenge for the multidisciplinary team. As mentioned earlier, ethical issues are important and the lack of accurate information on the pharmacokinetic behavior of chemotherapy in pregnant women is a serious technical obstacle [34, 40].

Constant fetal evaluation is required using cord blood samples (cordiocentesis) and ultrasounds because intrauterine exposure to chemotherapy drugs represents a significant risk of unfavorable outcomes such as low birth weight, fetal death, and intrauterine fetal death [38, 41].

1.7.2 Acute Promyelocytic Leukemia in Pregnancy

Acute promyelocytic leukemia is characterized by the presence of t-translocation (chromosomes 15 and 17) involving the retinoic acid receptor α (RAR-α) on Chromosome 17 and the promyelocytic leukemia gene on Chromosome 15. APL comprises about 5% of AML in the United States. In recent decades, anthracyclines, all-trans retinoic acids (ATRAs), and arsenic trioxide (ATO) have been used in the treatment of ALI with excellent long-term survival results proven in many studies [42–44].

The treatment of APL in pregnancy represents major challenges regarding the optimal management of the complications of the disease, as maternal and fetal well-being must be prioritized. It is considered that the thrombohemorragic and infectious risk may be higher during pregnancy, while the identification of differentiation syndrome may be more complicated. Diagnosis of APL in pregnancy is quite uncommon, and there is a lack of information on the treatment of early-onset APL during pregnancy. Even the non-systemic use of retinoids can lead to significant embryo/fetal teratogenicity, especially in the organogenesis phase, in the first trimester of pregnancy [45]. The clinical phenomenon of disseminated intravascular coagulation (ICD) often accompanies ALI; hence, sequelae of ICD in pregnant women are potentially threatening to both mother and fetus [46, 47].

Acute promyelocytic leukemia reaches higher proportions in young adults when compared to other types of AML. The average age of diagnosis is 47 years, which is much lower than the AML, that is, 66 years. Therefore, APL is more common in pregnancy than the other AML subtypes. However, there are other subtypes of AML more common than APL in the general population [48, 49].

It is very difficult to estimate the value definitively, but the number of acute leukemia cases is greater than the total number of chronic leukemia cases in pregnancy, similar to AML which is more common than lymphocytic leukemia in pregnancy [6, 50].

There is uncertainty about the pathogenesis of ALP differing from a pregnant woman to a nonpregnant woman. It is believed that there are hormonal and immunological changes during pregnancy that may create a state of cellular immunosuppression and inflammatory process, which may predispose to malignant diseases and alter the behavior of tumors [51, 52].

The diagnosis of ALI in the first trimester of pregnancy resulted in greater difficulties, with risks to the fetus and a high rate of spontaneity or therapeutic abortion, regardless of ATRA use. These findings show that current therapy is effective in pregnant women with ALI, but diagnosis and treatment may be associated with a high risk of obstetric and fetal complications. Until recently, the obstetric complications of APL therapy had been poorly understood, as they stemmed from individual case reports. Currently, it is possible to recognize high rates of fetal and obstetric complications in ALI, especially when the diagnosis occurs in the first trimester of pregnancy, regardless of the type of chemotherapy [53].

Patients diagnosed with APL during pregnancy represent an unusual challenge, requiring the approach of a hematologist, an obstetrician, and a neonatologist. But it is important to note that the treatment of APL depends essentially on the trimester of pregnancy in which the disease was diagnosed [56, 57].

The use of ATRA in the first trimester of pregnancy is associated with a high risk of teratogenicity and miscarriage [54]. The safety of anthracycline and cytarabine use has been well evaluated in some cases with follow-up. Use of cytarabine ($n = 93$) was associated with approximately 4% risk of limb malformations if used in the first trimester, 6% risk of intrauterine fetal death, 2% risk of neonatal mortality, and 13% of delayed intrauterine growth. Many of these adversities were noted with the combination of cytarabine with thioguanine and daunorubicin [55].

During the second and third trimesters of pregnancy, ATRA may be used, but arsenic-derived substances are contraindicated because they are highly embryotoxic [56, 57].

In women diagnosed with ALI in the second and third trimesters of pregnancy, the two main options available are as follows [56]:

1. Induction of ATRA remission only with postponement of chemotherapy administration until delivery.
2. Simultaneous administration of ATRA and chemotherapy as it is performed in nonpregnant women at the time of diagnosis.

Immediate administration of ATRA and chemotherapy provides the best chance of cure but is accompanied by an increased risk of miscarriage, prematurity, low birth weight, neonatal neutropenia, and sepsis; hence, induction of labor between cycles should be considered [56, 57]. Patients treated with ATRA alone, compared with patients treated with ATRA plus chemotherapy, have similar remission rates but higher rates of hyperleukocytosis and higher relapse rates. Patients treated with ATRA alone need continuous monitoring by RT-qPCR after remission induction to monitor for relapse pending delivery. Patients who are newly combined with ATRA and chemotherapy require strict fetal monitoring with a specific emphasis on cardiovascular functions [56, 57].

1.7.3   Acute Lymphoblastic Leukemia (ALL) in Pregnancy

Cervical and breast tumors are the most commonly diagnosed tumors during pregnancy, followed by melanoma, leukemia, and lymphoma. The treatment of malignancies during pregnancy has been updated, and the participation of the multidisciplinary team is important. Chemotherapy should be avoided during the first trimester as it has harmful effects on the fetus during the period of organogenesis. Even with the administration of chemotherapy during the second and third trimesters, there are cases of fetal growth restriction, intrauterine death and neonatal death, prematurity and myelosuppression [58].

Cases of ALL are relatively rare in adults: only 21 cases of this type of leukemia have been reported since 2009. Thus, there is little information and data about ALL, which precludes better recommendations for treatment during pregnancy [6, 7, 10].

The incidence of ALL is 1.3 per 100,000, with a slight male predominance. In nonpregnant adults, the complete remission rate reaches 80% of cases. Approximately 40% of adults are cured by modern treatment strategies, which gives an average 10-year survival. In the last 20 years, there has been a significant technological advance and the basic principle of all treatments has been chemotherapy: induction, consolidation, and maintenance therapy [59].

In the first trimester of pregnancy, the teratogenic effects of chemotherapy may occur in the treatment of ALL [60]. In the second and third trimesters of pregnancy, chemotherapy can cause a greater number of stillbirths, growth retardation, prematurity at birth, and maternal and fetal myelosuppression. Treatment during pregnancy seems to have no impact on the child's future growth and development. However, much of the scientific literature deals with acute myeloblastic leukemia rather than ALL. In ALL patients, pancytopenia, sudden intrauterine death and severe eclampsia have been reported. Acute leukemia requires immediate treatment regardless of gestational period. Acute leukemia does not have its course altered by pregnancy, but the outcome is much worse if initiation of treatment is delayed. Pregnant women should receive doses similar to nonpregnant women and because of the high risk of teratogenic effects of chemotherapy in the treatment of leukemia in the first trimester, termination of pregnancy should be considered [55, 61–63].

The structural basis of ALL's remission induction regimens is based on the use of vinca alkaloids, anthracyclines, cytarabine, and steroids. Vinca alkaloids have no teratogenic effects. In a group of 28 reported cases of ALL treated with anthracyclines after the first trimester of pregnancy, 21 had no complications. Cytarabine may produce limb abnormalities if used in the first trimester. The Cytarabine treatment was reported in 88 cases in all trimesters, with 6 intrauterine fetal deaths and 2 neonatal deaths [55].

Acute lymphoblastic leukemia chemotherapy regimens include cytarabine, cyclophosphamide, L-asparaginase, anthracyclines, corticosteroids, and vincristine [6].

Different chemotherapy induction regimens are used to treat ALL worldwide. It is important to remember the degree of malignancy of this type of leukemia and the need for immediate initiation of treatment. In the same country, several schemes can be used, such as CALGB, CCG, and DFCI in the United States and FRALLE, LALA, and GRAALL protocols in France. These treatment regimens undergo total modification or replacement as new protocols emerge. Even with the development of various induction regimes, it is still not possible to claim that there is a better treatment for ALL. The drugs constituting these therapeutic regimens are basically the same with different doses and dosing schedules [64–66].

In recent years, more intensified ALL pediatric treatment regimens have been used in patients aged 15–40 years. This is because many studies have shown that adolescents and young adults treated with adult chemotherapy regimens performed worse compared to patients in the same age group treated with pediatric protocols.

Some cancer centers are currently treating patients with ALL between 1 and 50 years with the same chemotherapy protocols and incorporating new agents such as nelarabine and rituximab. Therefore different from AML, in ALL, the use of different treatment regimens makes it difficult to adopt strong recommendations or even to establish strict guidelines for the treatment of ALL in pregnancy [64, 65, 67, 68].

The risk of congenital malformations is reduced as pregnancy progresses. There is a lack of information on autopsies performed on fetuses, as well as on malformations found [10]. The use of high-dose methotrexate is a crucial component in most ALL intensification protocols; however, the drug is highly teratogenic and its use during the first trimester of pregnancy is directly related to the development of aminopterin syndrome and a high risk of abortion [6, 7, 10].

The second trimester of pregnancy can be divided into two stages: first stage, before the 20th week of pregnancy. Management resembles the first trimester of pregnancy; hence, termination of pregnancy should be considered, followed by administration of appropriate or standard ALL induction therapy. In the second stage, that is, after the 20th week of gestation, bridge chemotherapy or ALL protocols without methotrexate may be administered until the third trimester of pregnancy, although damage to the fetus should be considered. Many regimens without methotrexate have been tested, but experience with these modified therapies is extremely limited; hence, these therapeutic regimens should be used as short-bridge treatments until the third trimester [6, 7, 10].

The frequency of acute leukemia in pregnancy is 1 in 750,000 cases and ALL represents between 11% and 28% of leukemia cases in pregnancy [58, 69]. Nevertheless, with ALL being rare in pregnancy, it can be quickly fatal if left untreated. Therefore, it requires immediate therapy regardless of gestational age [69, 70]. Many advances in the treatment of leukemia have provided survival and emphasized the importance of starting treatment before delivery. Many reported cases have been successful in treating ALL in pregnancy using many combinations of cytotoxic agents: prednisolone, cytarabine, cyclophosphamide, vincristine, daunorubicin or doxorubicin, L-asparaginase, 6-mercaptopurine, and intrathecal methotrexate [69].

However, the choice of the specific chemotherapy regimen depends on the gestational age and clinical condition of the pregnant woman, as well as the predicted toxicity events in the cytotoxic agents [69].

1.7.4   Chronic Myeloid Leukemia (CML) in Pregnancy

Chronic myeloid leukemia is a chronic myeloproliferative neoplasm characterized by reciprocal translocation between the long arms of chromosomes 9:22 t (9:22) (q34, q11), which results in a mutation in the *BCR-ABL* fusion gene that encodes a protein with tyrosine kinase. Currently, the standard model for treating this type of leukemia is tyrosine kinase inhibitors (TKIs). CML can occur in women of childbearing age, meaning that pregnancy can occur at diagnosis or during treatment with CML. Rarely will the diagnosis of CML happen during pregnancy. Management of this situation is changing due to the potent side effects of tyrosine kinase inhibitors (TKIs) on mother and fetus, with increased placental failure, low birth weight, increased prematurity, and perinatal morbidity and mortality. TKIs are potentially teratogenic and therefore not recommended during pregnancy. We know very little about the toxicity of TKIs in human embryos [76], but there are cases with good results in this type of treatment [71–77].

The hydroxyurea, interferon and leukapheresis are considered safe in patients with hyperleukocytosis. The use of TKIs in CML is not recommended due to the risk of pathogenicity and should be started as soon as possible before delivery. There are some cases where TKIs can be used but this will depend on the risk of the disease. Patients wishing to conceive even under TKI treatment should be advised to discontinue TKIs. This suspension should be made after achieving major molecular response (MMR) [78] or better responses and sustaining these responses for at least 2 years [10, 79, 80].

Imatinib should be taken shortly before ovulation and probably at the beginning of menstruation. The duration of discontinuation of imatinib therapy is limited to 6 months, but if the results of RT-qPCR analysis of BCR-ALB transcripts show no change (increase) from baseline, there may be an increase of the duration of the interruption. RT-qPCR and blood count should be monitored every 3 months while awaiting therapy with imatinib [10, 79].

We may consider replacing imatinib therapy with other therapeutic strategies such as leukapheresis, interferon and hydroxyurea; hence, the idea that, if necessary, interruption of imatinib therapy in CML pregnant women is of high risk [80–82].

There are very limited therapeutic experiences reported in the treatment of CML in pregnant women using dasatinib and nilotinib. In these studies, three miscarriages and four successful pregnancies were observed in dasatinib-treated CML pregnant women. In the same research group, a patient with CML diagnosed during pregnancy, treated with dasatinib was included, but unfortunately, she developed serious complications that led to termination of pregnancy [83, 84].

The use of leukapheresis in pregnant women with CML has been successful if used in the first trimester of pregnancy [10, 85, 86]. There is only one record of a myelomeningocele newborn who received leukapheresis and hydroxyurea during pregnancy [10].

1.7.5 Chronic Lymphocytic Leukemia in Pregnancy

Chronic lymphocytic leukemia (CLL) rarely occurs during pregnancy with few cases described in the literature; yet, it is the most common leukemia in the Western world [87, 88]. The average diagnosis of this disease is 72 years, and only 10% of all patients with CLL are below 55 years [89].

The most common complications of CLL in pregnant women are autoimmune phenomena, anemia requiring blood transfusions, hyperleukocytosis, and repeated infections [87].

Treatment strategies in CLL at any stage of pregnancy include leukapheresis for hyperleukocytosis, corticosteroids for autoimmune hemolytic anemia and autoimmune thrombocytopenia, and some antimicrobials for infectious complications of CLL [6, 7, 86].

When cancer is diagnosed during pregnancy or when pregnancy occurs after the diagnosis of cancer, many problems arise. No matter what the stage of the disease, it is important that pregnant women and their families receive the available information including therapeutic alternatives and fetal risks. Medical, emotional, behavioral, cultural, and family issues can affect choices, the final treatment decision. The decision involves not only the oncologist and the patient but the family as well. The inclusion of the multidisciplinary team helps clarify the picture, so that the best decision can be made [90].

Rituximab in the treatment of CLL in pregnancy and lactation is not recommended, because it is a drug authorized for use by the Food Drug Administration (FDA) as category C posing high risk when used in pregnancy. It has the potential to delay B cell reconstitution, with the effects being maintained for months or years after use. If possible, pregnancy should be delayed during treatment and even for 12 months after administration in pregnant women with CLL. There are reports of cases of neonatal lymphopenia and / or B cell depletion due to exposure to rituximab during pregnancy [91, 92].

A review article that followed 231 pregnancies associated with the use of rituximab found that there were 90 live births, 22 of them premature. One newborn died in the 6th week from unknown causes, even with pregnancy occurring 14 weeks after the use of rituximab. In this case, it should be noted that the pregnancy was complicated by the presence of systemic lupus erythematosus, gestational diabetes, and exposure to warfarin and prednisone [91].

Cladribine, a purine analogue drug, is active in LLC [93]. It reduces the rate of circulating CD4 T lymphocytes, leading to immune suppression, which may be exacerbated by pregnancy status. This is a category D drug with positive evidence of risk as teratogenic effects have been observed in animals. There are no data on the use of this drug with teratogenicity in humans yet. Cladribine antimetabolites are teratogenic and their use in pregnancy should be avoided. The same risks are observed when using fludarabine [6].

Chlorambucil should not be used during the first trimester of pregnancy as it has teratogenic effects, while fludarabine should not be used in pregnancy but may be used to treat CLL after delivery. During the second and third trimesters of pregnancy, the following medications can be safely used: rituximab, chlorambucil, and cyclophosphamide [7].

1.7.6   Hairy Cell Leukemia (HCL) in Pregnancy

The Hairy cell leukemia (HCL) has been recognized by the World Health Organization (WHO) since 2008 [94] and also included in the WHO review of the classification of lymphoid neoplasms [95]. HCL is more common in men than women (4–5 times), accounting for 2% of all leukemias, with approximately 1000 reported cases in the United States each year. HCL should be differentiated from other HCL-type pathologies including variant hairy cell leukemia (HCL-V) and diffuse red-fleshed splenic lymphoma (SDRPL) [96].

It is a very rare malignant disease in young women, especially pregnant women. If HCL is diagnosed during pregnancy, treatment will depend on whether or not pregnancy is terminated. If pregnancy is not interrupted or treatment is delayed until delivery, the following therapeutic options are possible: splenectomy, interferon, cladribine, rituximab, and other therapeutic modalities. Accurate diagnosis and detailed analysis are essential because the clinical profile of HCL can closely mimic that of other chronic B-cell lymphoproliferative disorders that are treated differently. The main indications for treatment are symptomatic cytopenias or painful splenomegaly. If a patient is asymptomatic and cytopenias are minimal, it is reasonable to adopt a watch-and-wait policy. It should be noted that the risk of opportunistic infections in patients with monocytopenia, with or without neutropenia, is high, precisely because of this reason, monitoring the evolution of clinical signs is of great importance [6, 7, 99–101].

The initial steps for hair cell recognition are complete blood counts and careful review of blood smears. HCL has an immunophenotypic profile characterized by clonal expansion of CD19, CD20, CD22, and CD200 B cells. Hair cells are generally negative for CD5, CD23, CD10, CD79b, and CD27, but positive for CD11c, CD103, CD123, and CD25 [97]. The treatment of HCL is based on the use of cladribine or pentostatin, but no randomized trials comparing pentostatin and cladribine have been reported. Moreover, there is no record in the literature about the superiority of either drug. In a large US database including 749 patients with HCL, cladribine was used in more than 75% of patients requiring first-line treatment [98]. If HCL infection cannot be controlled, interferon alfa may be an alternative in pregnant women. Combinations of fludarabine or bendamustine with rituximab have recently been explored in two small series with promising results, which projects possibility as an alternative therapy for HCL [101–103].

References

1. Slade R, James DK. Pregnancy and maternal malignant hematological disorders. In: Turner TL, editor. Perinatal hematological problems. Chichester: Wiley; 1991. p. 23–38.
2. Rothman LA, Cohen CJ, Astarloa J. Placental and fetal involvement by maternal malignancy: a report of rectal carcinoma and review of the literature. Am J Obstet Gynecol. 1973;116:1023–33.

3. Ewing PA, Whittaker JA. Acute leukemia in pregnancy. Obstet Gynecol. 1973;42:245–51.
4. Nicholson HO. Leukemia in pregnancy. Clin Obstet Gynecol. 1974;17:185–94. https://doi.org/10.1097/00003081-197412000-00013.
5. Greenlund LIS, Letendre L, Tefferi A. Acute leukemia during pregnancy: a single institution experience with 17 cases. Leuk Lymphoma. 2001;41:571–7. https://doi.org/10.3109/10428190109060347.
6. Shapira T, Pereg D, Lishner M. How I treat acute and chronic leukemia in pregnancy. Blood Rev. 2008;22:247–59.
7. Vandenbriele C, Vassou A, Pentheroudakis G, Van Calsteren K, Amant F. Hematologic malignancies in pregnancies. In: Actina M, editor. Acute leukemia-the scientist's perspective and challenge: InTech; 2011. ISBN: 978-953-307-553-2.
8. Seer Cancer Statistics Review [https://seer.cancer.gov.br]. StatFacts. Access in 01 Jan 2020. Available in https://seer.cancer.gov/statfacts/html/leuks.html.
9. Instituto Nacional de Câncer (INCA) [www.inca.gov.br]. Tipos de Câncer. 2018. Access in 01 Jan 2020. Available in https://www.inca.gov.br/tipos-de-cancer/leucemia.
10. Milojkovic D, Apperley JF. How I treat leukemia during pregnancy. Blood. 2014;123:974–84.
11. Mubara AA, Kakil IR, Awidi A, Al-Homsi U, Fawzi Z, et al. Normal outcome of pregnancy in chronic myeloid leukemia treated with interferón-alpha in 1st trimester report of 3 cases and review of the literatura. Am J Hematol. 2002;69(2):115–8.
12. Agarwal K, Patel M, Agarwal V. A complicated case of acute promyelocytic leukemia in the second trimester of pregnancy successfully treated with all-trans-retinoic acid. Case Rep Hematol. 2015;2015:634252.
13. Jacomo RH, Rego EM. Coagulation abnormalities in acute promyelocytic leukemia. Rev Bras Hematol Hemoter. 2009;31(2):48–50.
14. Giere I, Pavlovksy C, Van Thillo G. Planned pregnancy in a chronic myeloid leukemia patient in molecular remission. Case Rep Hematol. 2012;2012:624590.
15. Santiago-López CJ, Cuan-Baltazar Y, Pérez-Partida AM, Muñoz- Pérez MJ, Soto-Vega E. Leukemia During Pregnancy. Obstet Gynecol Int J. 2017;6(6):00225. https://doi.org/10.15406/ogij.2017.06.00225.
16. Ticku J, Oberoi S, Friend S, Busowski J, Langenstroer M, et al. Acute lymphoblastic leukemia in pregnancy: a case report with literature review. Ther Adv Hematol. 2013;4(5):313–9.
17. Pentheroudakis G. Cancer and pregnancy. Ann Oncol. 2008;19(5):38–9.
18. Conchon M, Sanabani S, Bendit I, Conchon M, Santos F, et al. Two successful pregnancies in a woman with chronic myeloid leukemia exposed to nilotinib during the first trimester of her second pregnancy: case study. J Hematol Oncol. 2009;2:42.
19. Matalon ST, Ornoy A, Fishman A, Drucker L, Lishner M. The effect of 6-mercaptopurine on early human placental explants. Hum Reprod. 2005;20(5):1390–7.
20. Moore KL. Embriologia Clinica. (10ª edición). Barcelona: Elsevier; 2016. p. 39–544.
21. Peccatori FA, Azim HA, Orecchia R, Hoekstra HJ, Pavlidis N, et al. Cancer, pregnancy and fertility: ESMO clinical practice guidelines for diagnosis, treatment and follow-up. Ann Oncol. 2013;24(suppl 6):vi160–70.
22. Saleh AJM, Alhejazi A, Ahmed SO, Al Mohareb F, AlSharif F, AlZahrani H, et al. Leukemia during pregnancy: long term follow up of 32 cases from a single institution. Hematol Oncol Stem Cell Ther. 2014;7(2):63–8.
23. Nomura RM, Igai AM, Faciroli NC, Aguiar IN, Zugaib M. Maternal and perinatal outcomes in pregnant women with leukemia. Rev Bras Ginecol Obstet. 2011;33(8):174–81.
24. Joydeb R, Maitreyee B, Kundu K, Madhavi P. Successful pregnancy outcome in a patient of chronic myeloid leukemia without therapy. J Obstet Gynecol India. 2011;61(5):565–6.
25. Amiwero CE, Izuegbuna OO, Olowosulu RO. Acute lymphoblastic leukaemia in pregnancy: a case report. Br J Med Res. 2014;4(21):3924–32.
26. Thomas X. Acute myeloid leukemia in the pregnant patient. Eur J Haematol. 2015;95(2):124–36.

27. Reynoso EE, Keating A, Baker MA. Acute leukemia occurring 19 years after treatment of acute lymphoblastic leukemia. Cancer. 1987;59(11):1963–5.
28. Weisz B, Meirow D, Schiff E, Lishner M. Impact and treatment of cancer during pregnancy. Expert Rev Anticancer Ther. 2004;4(5):889–902.
29. Gokal R, Durrant J, Baum JD, Bennett MJ. Successful pregnancy in acute monocytic leukaemia. Br J Cancer. 1976;34(3):299–302.
30. Pavanello F, Zucca E, Ghielmini M. Rituximab: 13 open questions after 20 years of clinical use. Cancer Treat Rev. 2016;53:38–46.
31. Benardete DN, Kershenovich J, Meraz D, Galnares JA, Olaya EJ. Uso de quimioterapia en el embarazo. Rev Med Inst Mex Seguro Soc. 2016;54(6):752–8.
32. Jemal A, Thomas A, Murray T, Thun M. Cancer estatistics 2002. CA Cancer J Clin. 2002;52:23.
33. Chang A, Patel S. Treatment of acute myeloid leukemia in pregnancy. Ann Pharmacother. 2015;49(1):48–68.
34. Jeelani S, Rasool J, Jan A, Sajad A, Khan JAA, Lone AR. Pregnancy with acute myeloid leukemia. Indian J Med Paediatr Oncol. 2008;29(4):47–8.
35. Yalcin AD, Aydemir N, Erbay H, Bir F. A case of acute myelomonocytic leukemia in a parturient whom refused the therapy. Internet J Hematol. 2003;l(1):1–4.
36. Biener DM, Gossing G, Kuehnl A, Cremer M, Dudenhausen JW. Diagnosis and treatment of maternal acute myeloid leukemia during pregnancy imitating HELLP syndrome. J Perinat Med. 2009;37(6):713–4.
37. Menezes J, Emerenciano M, Pimenta F, Filho GG, Magalhaes IQ, Saut' Ana M, et al. Occurrence of acute myeloid leukemia in young pregnant women. Clin Med Blood Dis. 2008;1:27–31.
38. Tashiro H, Umezawa K, Shirota M, Oka Y, Shirasaka R, Nishi R, et al. Acute myelogenous leukemia developed at the 26th week of gestation. Rinsho Ketsueki. 2011;52(11):18–22.
39. Larson RA. Induction therapy for acute myeloid leukemia in young adults. UpToDate 2014. Edited by Lowenberg B and Connor RF. Topic last updated: September 04, 2014.
40. Niedermeier DM, Frei-Lahr DA, Hall PD. Treatment of acute myeloid leukemia during the second and third trimesters of pregnancy. Pharmacotherapy. 2005;25(8):1134–40.
41. Morishita S, Imai A, Kawabata I, Tamaya T. Acute myelogenous leukemia in pregnancy. Fetal blood sampling and early effects of chemotherapy. Int J Gynecol Obstet. 1994;44(3):273–7.
42. Yamamoto JF, Goodman MT. Patterns of leukemia incidence in the United States by subtype and demographic characteristics, 1997–2002. Cancer Causes Control. 2008;19:379–90.
43. Ades L, Guerci A, Raffoux E, et al. Very long-term outcome of acute promyelocytic leukemia after treatment with all-trans retinoic acid and chemotherapy: the European APL Group experience. Blood. 2010;115:1690–6.
44. Lo-Coco F, Avvisati G, Vignetti M, et al. Retinoic acid and arsenic trioxide for acute promyelocytic leukemia. N Engl J Med. 2013;369:111–21.
45. D'Emilio A, Dragone P, De Negri G, et al. Acute myelogenous leukemia in pregnancy. Haematologica. 1989;74:601–4.
46. Franchini M, Di Minno MN, Coppola A. Disseminated intravascular coagulation in hematologic malignancies. Semin Thromb Hemost. 2010;36:388–403.
47. Tallman MS, Kwaan HC. Intravascular clotting activation and bleeding in patients with hematologic malignancies. Rev Clin Exp Hematol. 2004;8:E1.
48. Park JH, Qiao B, Panageas KS, et al. Early death rate in acute promyelocytic leukemia remains high despite all-trans retinoic acid. Blood. 2011;118:1248–54.
49. Dores GM, Devesa SS, Curtis RE, et al. Acute leukemia incidence and patient survival among children and adults in the United States, 2001–2007. Blood. 2012;119:34–43.
50. Thomas X. Acute myeloid leukemia in the pregnant patient . Eur J Haematol. 2015. https://doi.org/10.1111/ejh.12535. [Epub ahead of print].
51. Ioachim HL. Non-Hodgkin ' s lymphoma in pregnancy. Th ree cases and review of the literature. Arch Pathol Lab Med. 1985;109:803–9.

52. Shakhar K, Valdimarsdottir HB, Bovbjerg DH. Heightened risk of breast cancer following pregnancy: could lasting systemic immune alterations contribute? Cancer Epidemiol Biomark Prev. 2007;16:1082–6.
53. Verma V, Giri S, Manandhar S, Pathak R, Bhatt VR. Acute promyelocytic leukemia during pregnancy: a systematic analysis of outcome. Leuk Lymphoma. 2015:1–7. https://doi.org/1 0.3109/10428194.2015.1065977.
54. Lammer EJ, Chen DT, Hoar RM, et al. Retinoic acid embryopathy. N Engl J Med. 1985;313:837–41.
55. Cardonick E, Iacobucci A. Use of chemotherapy during human pregnancy. Lancet Oncol. 2004;5:283–91.
56. Larson RA. Initial treatment of acute promyelocytic leukemia in adults. UpToDate 2014. Edited by: Lowenberg B and Connor RF. Topic last updated: April 29, 2014.
57. Sanz MA, Grimwade D, Tallman MS, Lowenberg B, Fenaux P, Estey EH, et al. Management of acute promyelocytic leukemia: recommendation from an expert panel on behalf of the European Leukemia Net. Blood. 2009;113:1875–91.
58. Ticku J, Oberoi S, Friend S, Busowski J, Langenstroer M, Baidas S. Acute lymphoblastic leukemia in pregnancy: a case report with literature review. Ther Adv Hematol. 2013;4(5):313–9. https://doi.org/10.1177/2040620713492933.
59. Hoelzer D, Gokbuget N. Recent approaches in acute lymphoblastic leukemia in adults. Crit Rev Oncol Hematol. 2000;36:49–58.
60. Schaefer C. Drugs during pregnancy and lactation. Amsterdam: Elsevier Science; 2001.
61. Arnon J, Meirow D, Lewis-Roness H, Ornoy A. Genetic and teratogenic effects of cancer treatments on gametes and embryos. Hum Reprod Update. 2001;7:394–403.
62. Brell J, Kalaycio M. Leukemia in pregnancy. Semin Oncol. 2000;27:667–77.
63. Ebert U, Löffler H, Kirch W. Cytotoxic therapy and pregnancy. Pharmacol Ther. 1997;74:207–20.
64. Ribera J-M, Ribera J, Genesca E. Treatment of adolescents and young adults with acute lymphoblastic leukemia. Mediterr J Hematol Infect Dis. 2014;6(1):e2014052.
65. Larson RA. Induction therapy for Philadelphia chromosome negative acute lymphoblastic leukemia in adults. Up To Date; Topic 4524; Version 28.0; Topic edited by Lowenberg B, Connor RF. Topic last updated: December 23, 2014.
66. Rowe JM, Buck G, Burnett AK, Chopra R, Wiernik PH, Richards SM, et al. Induction therapy for adults with acute lymphoblastic leukemia: results of more than 1500 patients from the international ALL trial: MRC UKALL XII/ECOG E2993. Blood. 2005;106: 3760–7.
67. Nachman JB, La MK, Hunger SP, Heerema NA, Gaynon PS, Hastings C, et al. Young adults with acute lymphoblastic leukemia have an excellent outcome with chemotherapy alone and benefit from intensive postinduction treatment: a report from the Children's Oncology Group. J Clin Oncol. 2009;27(31):5189–94.
68. DeAngelo DJ. The treatment of adolescent and young adults with acute lymphoblastic leukemia. Hematology Am Soc Hematol Educ Program. 2005:123–30.
69. Bottsford-Miller J, Haeri S, Baker AM, Boles J, Brown MB-cell acute lymphocytic leukemia in pregnancy. Arch Gynecol Obstet. 2010. https://doi.org/10.1007/s00404-010-1647-2.
70. Molkenboer JFM, Vos AH, Shouten HC, Vos MC. Acute lymphoblastic leukemia in pregnancy. Neth J Med. 2005;63(5):361–3.
71. Mukhopadhyay A, Dasgupta S, Kanti Ray U, Gharami F, Bose CK, Mukhopadhyay S. Pregnancy outcome in chronic myeloid leukemia patient on imatinib therapy. Ir J Med Sci. 2015;184(1):183–8.
72. Hoffbrand AV, Moss PA. Fundamentos de hematologia. Editora Art Med 6 Cap. 2011;14(3):192–9.
73. Alizadeh H, Jaafar H, Rajnics P, Khan MI, Kajtár B. Outcome of pregnancy in chronic myeloid leukaemia patients treated with tyrosine kinase inhibitors: short report from a single center. Leuk Res. 2015;39(1):47–51.

74. Yadav U, Solanki SL, Yadav R. Chronic myeloid leukemia with pregnancy: successful management of pregnancy and delivery with hydroxyurea and imatinib continued till delivery. J Cancer Res Ther. 2013;9(3):484–6.
75. Apperley J. CML in pregnancy and childhood. Best Pract Res Clin Haematol. 2009;22(3):455–74.
76. Bayraktar S, Morency B, Escalón MP. Successful pregnancy in a patient with chronic myeloid leukaemia exposed to dasatinib during the first trimester. BMJ Case Rep. 2010;2010:bcr0520102975.
77. Conchon M, Sanabani SS, Benedit I, Santos FM, Serpa M, Dorliac-Llacer E. Two successful pregnancies in a woman with chronic myeloid leukemia exposed to nilotinib during the first trimester of her second pregnancy: case study. J Hematol Oncol. 2009;2:42.
78. de Moura AC, Delamain MT, Duarte GB, Lorand-Metze I, de Souza CA, Pagnano KB. Management of chronic myeloid leukemia during pregnancy: a retrospective analysis at a single center. Hematol Transfus Cell Ther. [Internet]. 2019 [cited 2020 Jan 09] ;41(2):125–128. Available from: http://www.scielo.br/scielo.php?script=sci_arttext&pid=S2531-13792019000200125&lng=en. Epub June 10, 2019. https://doi.org/10.1016/j.htct.2018.10.001.
79. Abruzzese E, Trawinska MM, Perrotti AP, De Fabritiis P. Tyrosine kinase inhibitors and pregnancy. Mediterr J Hematol Infect Dis. 2014;6(1):é2014028.
80. Usui N. Discontinuation of tyrosine kinase inhibitors and pregnancy for female patients with chronic myeloid leukemia. J Hematol Transfus. 2014;2(3):1023.
81. Negrin RS, Schiffer CA. Clinical use of tyrosine kinase inhibitors for chronic myeloid leukemia. UpToDate 2014. Edited by Larson RA and Connor RF. Topic last updated: October 22, 2014.
82. Pye SM, Cortes J, Ault P, Hatfield A, Kantarjian H, Pilot R, et al. The effects of imatinib on pregnancy outcome. Blood. 2008;111:5505–8.
83. Berveiller P, Andreoli A, Mir O, Anselem O, Delezoide AL, Sauvageon H, et al. A dramatic fetal outcome following transplacental transfer of dasatinib. Anti-Cancer Drugs. 2012;23(7):754–7.
84. Oweini H, Otrock ZK, Mahfouz RA, Bazarbachi A. Successful pregnancy involving a man with chronic myeloid leukemia on dasatinib. Arch Gynecol Obstet. 2011;283(1):133–4.
85. Klaasen R, de Jong P, Wijermans PW. Successful management of chronic myeloid leukemia with leukapheresis during a twin pregnancy. Neth J Med. 2007;65(4):147–9.
86. Ali R, Özkalemkas F, Özkocaman V, Özcelik T, Ozan U, Kimya Y, et al. Successful pregnancy and delivery in a patient with chronic myelogenous leukemia (CML) and management of CML with leukemia during pregnancy: a case report and review of the literature. Jpn J Clin Oncol. 2014;34(4):215–7.
87. Christomalis L, Baxi LV, Heller D. Chronic lymphocytic leukemia in pregnancy. Am J Obstet Gynecol. 1996;175:1381–2. https://doi.org/10.1016/S0002-9378(96)70062-5.
88. Hamad N, Kliman D, Best OG. Chronic lymphocytic leukaemia, monoclonal B-lymphocytosis and pregnancy: five cases, a literature review and discussion of management. Br J Haematol. 2014;68(3):350–60.
89. Eichhorst B, Dreyling M, Robak T, et al. ESMO Guidelines Working Group. Chronic lymphocytic leukemia: ESMO clinical practice guidelines for diagnosis, treatment and follow-up. Ann Oncol. 2011;22:50–4. https://doi.org/10.1093/annonc/mdr377.
90. Pereg D, Koren G, Lishner M. Cancer in pregnancy: gaps, challenges and solutions. Cancer Treat Rev. 2008;34:302–12. https://doi.org/10.1016/j.ctrv.2008.01.002.
91. Chakravarty EF, Murray ER, Farmer P. Pregnancy outcomes after maternal exposure to rituximab. Blood. 2011;117(5):1499–506. https://doi.org/10.1182/blood-2010-07-295444.
92. Klink DT, van Elburg RM, Schreurs MW, et al. Rituximab administration in third trimester of pregnancy suppresses neonatal B-cell development. Clin Dev Immunol. 2008;2008:271363. https://doi.org/10.1155/2008/271363.

93. CLL Trialists' Collaborative Group (CLLTCG). Systematic review of purine analog treatment for chronic lymphocytic leukemia: lessons for future trials. Hematologica. 2012;97(3):428–36. https://doi.org/10.3324/haematol.2011.053512.
94. Foucar K, Falini B, Catovsky D, Stein H. Hairy cell leukemia. In: Swerdlow SH, Campo E, Harris NL, editors. WHO classification of tumours of haematopietic and lymphoid tissues. Lyon: IARC Press; 2008.
95. Swerdlow SH, Campo E, Pileri SA, et al. The 2016 revision of the World Health Organization classification of lymphoid neoplasms. Blood. 2016;127(20):2375–90. https://doi.org/10.1182/blood-2016-01-643569.
96. Traverse-Glehen A, Baseggio L, Bauchu EC, et al. Splenic red pulp lymphoma with numerous basophilic villous lymphocytes: a distinct clinicopathologic and molecular entity? Blood. 2008;111(4):2253–60. https://doi.org/10.1182/blood-2007-07-098848.
97. Matutes E, Morilla R, Owusu-Ankomah K, Houliham A, Meeus P, Catovsky D. The immunophenotype of hairy cell leukemia (HCL). Proposal for a scoring system to distinguish HCL from B-cell disorders with hairy or villous lymphocytes. Leuk Lymphoma. 1994;14(Suppl 1):57–61.
98. Divino V, Karve S, Gaughan A, et al. Characteristics and treatment patterns among US patients with hairy cell leukemia: a retrospective claims analysis. J Comp Eff Res. 2017;6(6):497–508. https://doi.org/10.2217/cer-2017-0014.
99. Ainoon O, Megat R, Cheong SK, Halimah Y. Hairy cell leukemia: a case report. Med J Malaysia. 1988;43(1):62–4.
100. Bustamante A, Rodriguez MA, Ocqueteau M, Bertin P, Lira P, Valbuena J. Hairy cell leukemia during pregnancy: report of one case. Rev Med Chil. 2010;138(11):1422–6.
101. López-Rubio M, Garcia-Marco JA. Current and emerging treatment options for hairy cell leukemia. Onco Targets Ther. 2015;8:2147–56.
102. Gerrie AS, Zypchen LN, Connors JM. Fludarabine and rituximab for relapsed or refractory hairy cell leukemia. Blood. 2012;119(9):1988–91.
103. Burotto M, Stetler-Stevenson M, Arons E, Zhou H, Wilson W, Kreitman RJ. Bendamustine and rituximab in relapsed and refractory hairy cell leukemia. Clin Cancer Res. 2013;19(22):6313–21.
104. Al-Anazi. Update on leukemia in pregnancy. In: Guenova, Balatzenko (eds) Leukemias – updates and new insights. IntechOpen; 2015. https://doi.org/10.5772/61290. Available from: https://www.intechopen.com/books/leukemias-updates-and-new-insights/update-on-leukemia-in-pregnancy.

Chapter 2
Clinical Perspectives for Leukemia Treatment During Pregnancy

Giancarlo Fatobene, Ana Costa Cordeiro, Maria Cecília Borges Bittencourt, and Rafael Fernandes Pessoa Mendes

2.1 Introduction

It is estimated that 1:75,000 to 100,000 pregnancies are complicated with leukemia [1]. Acute myeloid leukemia (AML) is estimated to represent 40% of the leukemias diagnosed during pregnancy, followed by acute lymphoblastic leukemia (ALL) in 25% and chronic myeloid leukemia (CML) in 25% [2]. Leukemias can greatly impact the outcomes of pregnancy, but it depends on the type of leukemia, type of treatment required, and pregnancy stage (Fig. 2.1). In this chapter, we consider the first trimester as weeks 1–13, second trimester as weeks 14–27, and third trimester from week 28 up to the end of pregnancy.

2.2 Acute Leukemias

Acute leukemias include AML, ALL, and acute promyelocytic leukemia (APL). More than two-thirds of acute leukemias diagnosed during pregnancy are AML [3]. All acute leukemias are medical emergencies. They can rapidly lead to pancytopenia and coagulation abnormalities. Without timely, adequate treatment, patients succumb to bleeding, infection, and organ dysfunction within days to weeks.

Acute leukemias are also associated with poor fetal outcomes. Both placenta and fetus can be adversely affected by maternal conditions including anemia, poor

G. Fatobene (✉)
Hospital das Clínicas - University of São Paulo and Hospital Sírio-Libanês, São Paulo, Brazil

A. C. Cordeiro · M. C. B. Bittencourt
Centro Paulista de Oncologia and Hospital 9 de Julho, São Paulo, Brazil

R. F. P. Mendes
Hospital Sírio-Libanês, São Paulo, Brazil

© Springer Nature Switzerland AG 2021
C. W. P. Schmidt, K. M. Otoni (eds.), *Chemotherapy and Pharmacology for Leukemia in Pregnancy*, https://doi.org/10.1007/978-3-030-54058-6_2

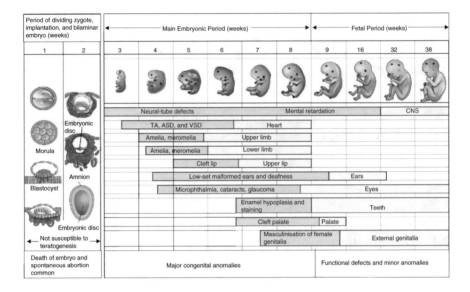

Fig. 2.1 Prenatal development. (Reproduced with permission from Moore P, ed. The developing human, 6th edition, 1998). Dots on the fetus indicate common sites of action of teratogenic agents. Horizontal bars show fetal development during highly sensitive period (purple) and less sensitive period (green). TA truncus arteriosus, ASD atrial septal defect, VSD ventricular septal defect

oxygen delivery, increased risk of bleeding, and thrombosis [4]. Although rare, there are cases of placenta involvement with leukemic cells [1] and vertical transmission of leukemia [5].

Chemotherapy, usually multiagent cytotoxic chemotherapy, is the only curative treatment for acute leukemias and should be started promptly [6]. However, it can be harmful to fetal tissues, especially during active organogenesis, mainly over weeks 3 and 10 of pregnancy [7]. Therefore, it is extremely important to have a reliable estimate of gestational age to decide the best medical approach.

The treatment of acute leukemias is divided into induction of remission, consolidation, and, depending on type of leukemia, maintenance. It differs for AML, APL, and ALL and is discussed separately in the next sections. Overall, there are no specific protocols for leukemia during pregnancy. Although some authors suggest dose reductions [8], doses are usually administered based on actual body weight [9, 10]. Pregnancy induces physiological changes in plasma volume and renal clearance in addition to third spacing (amniotic fluid), leading to a lower final serum concentration of drugs (discussed in Chaps. 4 and 5).

2.2.1 Considerations for the First Trimester

2.2.1.1 Miscarriages

The rate of miscarriage in pregnant women receiving chemotherapy for various malignancies is 20%, compared to 3–4% in the healthy population. Aviles et al. determined 23 of 216 (10.6%) acute leukemias diagnosed during the first trimester resulted in spontaneous abortion [11]. It is difficult to separate the effect of chemotherapy from acute leukemia itself. Miscarriages are risky for mothers due to pancytopenia, especially thrombocytopenia leading to bleeding. Spontaneous abortion and fetal death have been recurrently reported when patients decide not to undergo elective termination [12, 13]. In fact, intrauterine fetal demise or spontaneous abortion seem to be the most common outcomes of cytotoxic insult during the first trimester, rather than congenital malformations, which appears to be at lower risk than estimated [14–16].

2.2.1.2 Malformations

The rate of major congenital malformation in the general population reported in literature is between 5.1% and 6.9% [17]. Most studies on the effect of chemotherapy during the first trimester were not restricted to hematological malignancies. Doll et al. reported 139 cases of newborns exposed to multiagent chemotherapy (not restricted to hematological malignancies) in the first trimester, which showed malformations in 25% of newborns compared to 17% with single-agent chemotherapy [18]. If folate antagonists are excluded from this analysis, the rate of malformation with single-agent chemotherapy is 6% [19]. Cardonick et al. reported 376 cases receiving chemotherapy during pregnancy (any trimester) and found that 9 of 11 malformations observed were associated with chemotherapy in the first trimester [9]. Selig et al. reviewed 133 patients exposed to chemotherapy and showed 16%, 8%, and 6% of malformations in the first, second, and third trimesters, respectively. The rates of malformations were higher for alkylating agents (22%) and antimetabolites (15%), while vincristine was associated with low risks [14, 20]. On the other hand, Van Calsteren et al. studied 215 patients with various malignancies, including 26 treated with chemotherapy during the first trimester, and showed no increased risk of malformations [2].

In patients exclusively treated for hematological malignancies, Aviles et al. studied 58 newborns from mothers receiving intensive dose chemotherapy in the first trimester, including 14 for acute leukemias, and did not observe malformations [11]. They also reviewed the literature and showed that 16 of 216 (7.4%) acute leukemias diagnosed during the first trimester resulted in congenital malformations [11].

2.2.2 Considerations for the Second and Third Trimesters

Although eyes, genitalia, central nervous system, and hematopoietic cells are still vulnerable after the first trimester [19], many studies showed that chemotherapy in the second and third trimesters is not associated with malformations [9, 18]. However, it still carries fetal risks such as stillborn, intrauterine growth retardation, prematurity, low birthweight, and transient myelosuppression [3, 9, 14, 21]. Chemotherapy administered 3–4 weeks prior to delivery can induce hematological toxicity, placing mother and child in a vulnerable condition to infectious and bleeding complications during and after delivery [22], Thus, delaying elective deliveries for at least 3 weeks after the last dose of chemotherapy is recommended [14].

2.2.3 Clinical Recommendations for Acute Leukemias

Given the risk of miscarriages and malformations, it is reasonable to advise medical termination of pregnancy when acute leukemia is diagnosed in the first trimester [3, 23]. However, it is necessary to balance risks and family expectations (Fig. 2.2). If elective abortion is not acceptable to the mother but cure of the hematological malignancy is still considered reasonable, chemotherapy at full doses might be safe even during the first trimester, though there is a high potential for unintended fetal loss and malformations [14, 15].

With advances in neonatology, high rates of survival following early delivery are achieved. For the period between 24 and 35 weeks, risks and benefits of chemotherapy versus early delivery must be weighted on an individual basis. Chemotherapy protocol modification may be considered depending on gestational age [9].

Chemotherapy should not be given after 35–36 weeks of pregnancy [7, 9, 23]. At this stage, delivery is considered safe and with appropriate support, the newborn can be managed without increased risk.

For ethical reasons, fertility after chemotherapy (and possibly allogeneic stem cell transplantation) should be discussed with the patient before initiating oncological treatment.

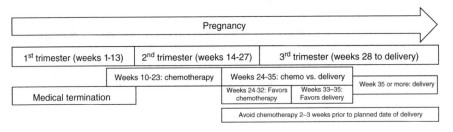

Fig 2.2 Summary of clinical approach for acute leukemias diagnosed during pregnancy

Hyperleukocytosis with leukostasis is a medical emergency. Leukapheresis can be used in pregnant women [24] but is generally not recommended for APL [25]. Hydroxyurea is only a palliative measure for acute leukemias, and we and others [23] recommend against its use during pregnancy for that indication.

2.2.4 Acute Myeloid Leukemia

Acute myeloid leukemia (AML) accounts for two-thirds of acute leukemias diagnosed during pregnancy [3, 7, 26, 27]. Leukemia risk stratification seems to be similar to nonpregnant women. Chelghoum et al. reviewed 37 cases of acute leukemia diagnosed during pregnancy, mostly AML, and found the proportion of favorable and normal karyotype to be similar to nonpregnant women [3].

Acute myeloid leukemia induction treatment is traditionally based on anthracyclines, usually daunorubicin or idarubicin × 3 days plus cytarabine as a continuous infusion × 7 days ("3+7" regimen). In one study, 58% of women diagnosed with AML during pregnancy received 3+7 therapy [28].

Daunorubicin and doxorubicin seem safe even in the first trimester of pregnancy. Idarubicin is more lipophilic and can cross the placenta easily [9]; hence, it has a higher probability of causing adverse effects in the fetus. There are some reports of fetal cardiomyopathy associated with idarubicin [9, 29–31].

Doxorubicin is widely used for breast cancer, including during pregnancy. Some authors suggest using doxorubicin in AML because it has been studied more in pregnant women [32–35], while others consider daunorubicin the anthracycline of choice in pregnancy [31, 35, 36].

One study including nonpregnant individuals compared doxorubicin 30 mg/m² versus daunorubicin 30 or 45 mg/m² × 3 days, both in combination with cytarabine 100 mg/m² × 7 days in continuous infusion, and showed that doxorubicin was more toxic and inferior in inducing complete remission (CR) than daunorubicin [37]. On the other hand, one study compared doxorubicin 45 mg/m² and idarubicin 12 mg/m² × 3 days, both in combination with cytarabine 100 mg/m² × 7 days continuous infusion and found similar complete remission (CR) and adverse event rates in both groups [38]. The National Comprehensive Cancer network (NCCN) guidelines do not include doxorubicin for AML treatment [25].

Cytarabine has been associated with limb malformations [18], and thus, it is reasonable to avoid it during organogenesis. If the patient requires AML treatment before 10 weeks of pregnancy, risks and benefits of anthracycline and cytarabine need to be discussed. We recommend avoiding cytarabine before 10 weeks of pregnancy due to the risk of malformation [39–41]. In this situation, treatment with anthracycline only (daunorubicin or doxorubicin) may be considered when the patient refuses pregnancy termination, but it is important to highlight the potential adverse effect of this strategy on AML prognosis.

There are many reports of successful outcomes in pregnant women treated with induction based on anthracyclines and cytarabine for AML during the second and third trimesters [3, 6, 26, 28, 36]. Ali et al. recommended daunorubicin 60 mg/m^2 on days 1, 3, and 5 plus cytarabine 100 mg/m^2 b.i.d. for 10 days [23], but 7 days of cytarabine is the standard and most commonly regimen used for AML. Since there is likely a benefit from using daunorubicin 90 mg/m^2 versus 45 mg/m^2 [42] and the fact that physiological changes during pregnancy lead to a lower final serum concentration of drugs, we recommend daunorubicin 90 mg/m^2 associated with cytarabine 100 mg/m^2 continuous infusion × 7 days (doses based on actual body weight) for pregnant women after 10 weeks of pregnancy. Novel drugs for AML in first-line therapy such as FLT3 and IDH inhibitors have not been studied in pregnant women, and thus, we do not recommend their use in this setting unless medical termination of pregnancy is pursued.

The median time from diagnosis to treatment in pregnant women has been reported to be only 6 days [3] and 65% received therapy within 1 week of diagnosis [28]. CR is attained in 71% of pregnant women undergoing AML treatment irrespective of the trimester of diagnosis, but it is higher (91%) in patients receiving standard anthracycline- and cytarabine-based treatment. Conversely, overall survival was lower in patients who had a delay in induction and consolidation treatment and/or received lower doses of chemotherapy [28].

Delivery after recovery from induction chemotherapy is recommended. If delivery is not possible due to gestational age, we recommend consolidation therapy with high-dose cytarabine, although there are no data available [43]. Reinduction with the same 3+7 regimen should be discussed on an individual basis. For refractory disease, we recommend termination of pregnancy to allow intensive chemotherapy and expedite allogeneic hematopoietic stem cell transplant.

2.2.5 Acute Promyelocytic Leukemia

Acute promyelocytic leukemia is characterized by translocation between chromosomes 15 and 17, resulting in the *PML-RARA* fusion gene. It differs from other AML types because it is associated with marked coagulopathy and considered a medical emergency. Delays in initiating APL treatment are associated with high morbidity and mortality. Transfusion support is extremely important and is discussed in the supportive therapy section. APL patients with white blood cell count (WBC) > 10,000/mm^3 are considered at high risk for complications and relapse.

The preferred regimens for APL induction of remission include all-trans retinoic acid (ATRA) plus arsenic trioxide (ATO) or idarubicin (at higher doses than previously described for AML) [25]. ATO is embryotoxic and contraindicated at all pregnancy stages [44].

All-trans retinoic acid is a retinoic acid belonging to the same family of isotretinoin. Isotretinoin is classically associated with major fetal malformations [45]. As such, ATRA is also associated with fetal malformations and spontaneous abortion in the first trimester but is safe during the second and third trimesters [4, 46–48].

All APL patients diagnosed early in the first trimester should be offered medical termination of pregnancy. For patients in the first trimester with marked coagulopathy and/or leukostasis, delays in initiating ATRA can dramatically increase the risks for the mother, and in this particular situation, therapeutic abortion is highly advisable [44, 49]. If the patient chooses termination of pregnancy, standard treatment with ATRA and chemotherapy should be initiated immediately to allow coagulation normalization to perform the abortion [44]. For patients in the first trimester who refuse pregnancy termination, treatment with anthracycline only (daunorubicin or doxorubicin) should be considered and ATRA could be added from the second trimester forward [44, 50]. However, it is important to highlight the potential adverse effect of this strategy on APL prognosis [51].

For APL patients diagnosed in the second and third trimesters of pregnancy, there are three strategies: (1) ATRA monotherapy; (2) ATRA + idarubicin (LPA 99 trial, also called AIDA regimen); and (3) ATRA + daunorubicin + cytarabine (APL 2000 trial).

Treatment with ATRA monotherapy increases the risk of differentiation syndrome (DS), especially for patients with WBC > 10,000/L [52, 53]. DS is characterized by a systemic inflammatory response, with capillary leak and leukostasis beginning days to weeks after treatment with ATRA and/or ATO [52]. Steroids can be used to prevent or treat DS. Prophylactic steroids are indicated in high-risk patients (WBC > 5000–10,000/mm^3) [25, 52]. If the decision is to use ATRA monotherapy for a prolonged period, *PML-RARA* should be monitored due to the increased risk of resistance and relapse [54, 55].

Idarubicin is not the anthracycline of choice during pregnancy (as discussed in the previous section) and its dose is higher for APL than for other types AML. Nevertheless, Sanz et al. reported successful outcomes for APL treated with ATRA plus idarubicin later in pregnancy (mostly >30 weeks) [56]. Special attention should be paid to the fetus due to the risk of fetal cardiac toxicity [29].

In nonpregnant women, AIDA showed a lower cumulative incidence of relapse (CIR) in patients with low risk, while APL 2000 regimen showed higher incidence of CR, overall survival, and a trend toward lower cumulative incidence of relapse in patients with high-risk APL [57].

Although ATRA can be used as monotherapy or short bridge to delivery [58], we favor treatment with ATRA plus chemotherapy [44]. Accordingly, we recommend the use of APL 2000 (ATRA + daunorubicin + cytarabine) in the second and third trimesters, irrespective of APL risk, due to the fetal risks that have been linked to idarubicin. However, AIDA (ATRA + idarubicin) is a reasonable choice for low-risk APL in third trimester.

Verma et al. [49] reported 71 APL cases diagnosed during pregnancy, 42% of whom received induction with ATRA + anthracyclines; 23% with ATRA monotherapy; and 13% with ATRA, anthracycline, and cytarabine. The CR rate was 93.1% for the whole population. Even though there were higher rates of obstetrical and fetal complications in the first trimester compared with the second and third trimesters, no significant difference was found according to the type of chemotherapy or inclusion of ATRA.

Delivery after recovery from induction chemotherapy is recommended. If delivery is not possible due to gestational age, we recommend a consolidation cycle using the same drugs of induction. After delivery, consolidation therapy can be intensified with ATO. If the disease is refractory, we recommend pregnancy termination and an ATO-based containing regimen.

2.2.6 Acute Lymphoblastic Leukemia

Approximately one-third of acute leukemia cases diagnosed in association with pregnancy is ALL [3, 12, 59]. The disease course is not altered nor has different outcomes purely because of the pregnant state [12, 59, 60]. Due to the rarity of ALL in pregnancy, there are no guidelines to direct its treatment; thus, optimal management recommendations are taken from case reports and small retrospective series, most of which also include AML data [3, 12, 14, 33, 59, 61]. Among pregnant women with ALL, most cases are of B-cell origin, but T-cell ALL has also been reported [62, 63]. Newly diagnosed ALL is more common during pregnancy than relapsed disease, though there have been a few cases reported [63–66].

Young adults diagnosed with ALL may be treated with either pediatric or adult protocols. Evidence favors pediatric-based protocols in view of improved event-free and overall survival [59]. Most induction regimens consist of a pre-phase with steroids, followed by a combination of four or five drugs: daunorubicin, cyclophosphamide, vincristine, and steroids with or without asparaginase [3]. Intrathecal cytarabine, methotrexate, and hydrocortisone are also part of different protocols [14]. Other drugs commonly used during consolidation and maintenance include systemic cytarabine and methotrexate, as well as 6-mercaptopurine. Hyper-CVAD, an adult protocol commonly used for the treatment of ALL, incorporates doxorubicin instead of daunorubicin and does not include asparaginase and 6-mercaptopurine [21, 67]. This regimen is often used for chromosome Philadelphia-positive (Ph+) ALL [68, 69]. Although it has not been widely used for pregnant women, it has been reported by some groups [21, 67]. GRAAPH, a reduced-intensity protocol for Ph+ ALL (without anthracycline), has not yet been reported in pregnant patients [70].

2.2.6.1 Considerations for Protocol Adjustments in Pregnant Women

Most studies advocate using standard treatments without adjustments of protocol-directed doses [12, 14, 59, 60, 71, 72]. However, some modifications have been reported. For instance, later in the third trimester, some ALL patients were offered only vincristine and prednisone to control of the disease before delivery [60, 71]. Considering the myelosuppression caused by anthracyclines and the consequent risk of sepsis, daunorubicin was left out in a study, despite its association with superior complete remission rates [73]. Maintenance was also used instead of consolidation to avoid cytopenias related with cyclophosphamide [73]. Methotrexate and asparaginase, crucial components of most protocols of ALL, have also been omitted [13].

Methotrexate is highly teratogenic at doses greater than 10 mg per week in the first trimester. It has been associated with an increased risk of cranial dysostosis, delayed ossification, hypertelorism, wide nasal bridge, micrognathia, and ear anomalies (aminopterin syndrome) [9, 14]. As a category X drug, its use is not advised during pregnancy, particularly before 28 weeks of gestation, although it may be used with caution in the third trimester [67, 74]. Exposure during the second and third trimesters, including intrathecal infusions, has been reported without deleterious outcomes [14, 60, 67, 68]. However, it has most frequently been postponed until after delivery or completely eliminated [14, 21, 22, 73, 75].

Asparaginase is one of the main risk factors for the occurrence of venous thromboembolism in ALL as it decreases the levels of thrombotic inhibitors, such as antithrombin III [76]. Pregnancy is a hypercoagulable state per se with increased risk of thrombosis during gestation and puerperium [14, 22, 59]. Cesarean delivery further raises its likelihood [13]. Therefore, asparaginase should be avoided throughout pregnancy, unless the expected benefit outweighs the risks [13, 59]. Prophylactic low-molecular-weight heparin (LMWH) is safe in pregnant patients, and despite the limited data, it is recommended during treatment with asparaginase if there is no contraindication [14, 76–78]. LMWH at therapeutic doses until 6 weeks postpartum was described in a case report to allow treatment with full doses of asparaginase and steroids [22]. Hypofibrinogenemia and bleeding are other undesirable side effects of asparaginase [21, 76–78]; thus, clinical benefit of LMWH must be weighed against the bleeding risk [76–78]. Supplementing antithrombin III has also been recommended to maintain plasma levels above 50–60% during asparaginase treatment [76, 78]. Antithrombin III replacement and prophylactic LMWH have been used either alone or in combination [77, 78]. Pancreatitis, another possible adverse effect of asparaginase, is usually subclinical and resolves after cessation of the drug, but insulin synthesis inhibition and glutamine metabolism disorders may induce hyperosmolar hyperglycemia [22, 77]. Close monitoring of patients on insulin therapy is recommended after discontinuation of asparaginase in order to avoid hypoglycemia induced by normalized endogenous insulin synthesis [77]. Although there is no need for dose adjustment, steroids used in the induction phase add risk to both venous thromboembolism and hyperglycemia in the context of pregnancy and treatment with asparaginase [22, 76]. Due to these adverse effects, asparaginase administration requires monitoring of the coagulation system, hepatic and pancreatic enzymes, and glucose levels [78].

2.2.6.2 Chromosome Philadelphia (Ph+)-Positive ALL

The translocation involving the chromosomes 9 and 22 (known as Philadelphia [Ph] chromosome) is found in 15–30% of adults with ALL [67]. This rearrangement, t(9;22)(q34;q11), generates a fusion gene called *BCR-ABL1*, which codes for a p190 or, less commonly, p210 BCR-ABL1 oncoprotein with high tyrosine kinase activity [79]. Tyrosine kinase inhibitors (TKIs) in combination with chemotherapy are currently the standard therapy for Ph+ ALL in the general adult population [80, 81]. Five tyrosine kinase inhibitors are under clinical use nowadays: first-generation imatinib; second-generation nilotinib, dasatinib, and bosutinib; and third-generation ponatinib. Even though the best chemotherapy regimen to be administered with TKIs remains unknown, combinations with Hyper-CVAD and GRAAPH are described [81].

A large international retrospective study evaluated 180 women with various hematologic malignancies exposed to imatinib during pregnancy, 71% in the first trimester [82]. Among the 125 cases with known outcomes, 63 pregnancies (50%) resulted in normal live births, 35 (28%) underwent elective terminations, and 18 (14.4%) ended in spontaneous abortion, slightly higher than the spontaneous abortion rate of 10–12% in the normal population. Twelve infants (9.6%) were reported to have congenital malformations and ten of them were known to be exposed to imatinib during the first trimester. The fetal abnormalities included premature closure of skull sutures (craniosynostosis), hypoplastic lungs, duplex kidney, absent kidney, shoulder anomaly, exomphalos, renal agenesis, hemivertebrae, and scoliosis.

A pharmacovigilance database review [83] reported pregnancy outcomes available in 46 out of 78 women treated with dasatinib. Fifteen pregnancies (33%) resulted in deliveries of normal infants at term, although dasatinib was discontinued in 12 of these 15 women in the first trimester. Five pregnancies (11%) were abnormal because of placental complications or prematurity but resulted in live births. Elective or spontaneous abortions occurred in 18 (39%) and 8 (17%) women, respectively. Seven fetal abnormalities were reported, including hydrops fetalis, lung hypoplasia, and renal tract and CNS abnormalities. Placental transfer of dasatinib has been described [83, 84], which discourages its use at any time during pregnancy.

The experience with nilotinib during pregnancy is rather small, based only on case reports [85]. Although some successful pregnancies have been described in women receiving nilotinib, safety evidence is still limited. Unlike dasatinib, nilotinib does not significantly cross the placental barrier. Regarding bosutinib and ponatinib, there are no consistent data available; thus, these agents should not be considered during pregnancy.

Even though evidence supports initiation of TKIs together with chemotherapy in the treatment of Ph+ ALL in the general population [67, 81], this may not be as straightforward in pregnant patients [67]. As serious abnormalities may have occurred with exposure to TKIs in the first trimester, we strongly suggest elective termination in case Ph+ ALL is diagnosed at this point [21, 61, 67, 82, 86]. Even later in gestation TKIs might not be free of risks [74, 83]. Since CR rates of 60–70% can still be expected when TKIs are not used in the induction phase for ALL, this drug class should be avoided until after delivery if possible [22, 61].

When considering pregnancy in patients who have achieved major molecular response and are on long-term maintenance, TKI therapy may be safely interrupted and the patients placed on interferon therapy, starting 2 months before cessation of oral contraceptives throughout pregnancy [80].

2.2.6.3 Other Drugs

Newer target therapy drugs for ALL include nelarabine for ALL-T and blinatumumab and inotuzumab ozogamicin for ALL-B. Their use during pregnancy has not yet been reported in the literature. Rituximab has been added to the treatment of CD20-positive ALL with improved event-free survival and overall survival [81]. Nonetheless, pregnant women were not included in the studies, and there are some concerns with the use of rituximab during pregnancy, as it may cause premature birth, neonatal infection, lymphopenia, and/or B-cell depletion [87, 88].

2.3 Chronic Leukemias

Chronic leukemias are diseases characterized by the accumulation of differentiated cells (myeloid or lymphoid) in the peripheral blood. In contrast with acute leukemias, they are usually indolent diseases that may not require immediate treatment and can be managed with watchful waiting. Median ages at diagnosis of CML and chronic lymphocytic leukemia (CLL) are 66 and 70 years, respectively [89, 90], but a few patients may be diagnosed at reproductive age. Hairy cell leukemia (HCL) is another chronic leukemia that is rare at reproductive age. The most common scenario in this setting is a young woman previously diagnosed with CML or CLL who wants to get pregnant. Counselling in this situation is extremely important. Patients who have been treated and are willing to get pregnant need information regarding the risk of disease progression during pregnancy and the potential side effects of treatment on the fetus [91]. Chronic leukemias requiring prompt treatment are rarely diagnosed during pregnancy.

2.3.1 Chronic Myeloid Leukemia

Chronic myeloid leukemia (CML) is a distinctive myeloproliferative neoplasm characterized by a balanced genetic translocation between chromosomes 9 and 22, which results in the p210 BCR-ABL fusion protein. CML is responsible for approximately 15% of newly diagnosed cases of leukemia in adults, with an overall incidence of 1–2 cases per 100,000 [92]. CML is more common among older adults but can occur in all age groups. Actually, at least one-quarter of patients will be at reproductive age at diagnosis, and this proportion may be even higher in countries with younger populations [86, 93, 94].

Most patients present in chronic phase (CP) and are usually asymptomatic. However, if not properly treated, the disease may progress to accelerated (AP) and blast (BP) phases, ultimately evolving to acute leukemia, with anemia, bleeding, and infectious complications. Until 2000, limited therapies were available for CML, including hydroxyurea and interferon-alfa, and allogeneic hematopoietic stem cell transplantation was the only treatment able to provide long-term remission. However, after the development of TKIs, survival in CML patients has dramatically improved, achieving similar life expectancy as the general population [95].

2.3.1.1 Drug Selection in Pregnancy

As discussed previously, TKIs are to be avoided in pregnancy, particularly during embryogenesis in the first trimester. CML management during pregnancy is not defined in current guidelines. Different from Ph+ ALL whose treatment with TKIs during pregnancy is more pressing, many reports have investigated alternative therapies to TKIs capable of controlling CP CML until childbirth [86, 93, 96].

Hydroxyurea, a cytotoxic agent which inhibits DNA synthesis, is not recommended during pregnancy as it has teratogenic potential apart from its limited efficacy in CML. Hydroxyurea use has been implicated in intrauterine deaths, congenital malformations, premature births, and higher incidence of preeclampsia in the second and third trimesters [86, 96, 97].

The most common alternative to treat CML during pregnancy is interferon-alfa (IFN-α). It has been extensively used in clinical practice before the advent of TKIs. Although not prone to providing deep responses, IFN-α has a modest action against the malignant CML clone through its effects on protein synthesis, RNA breakdown, and immunomodulation. Owing to its high molecular weight, it does not cross the placenta and is not teratogenic [86, 96, 97].

The side effects caused by IFN-α sometimes may be difficult to tolerate, including flu-like symptoms, myelosuppression, fatigue, and depression. Nonetheless, many studies have demonstrated its safety during pregnancy. A systematic review compiled 63 case reports of pregnancies exposed to IFN-α and showed only one case of spontaneous abortion and no stillbirths or fetal malformations [98].

An alternative is leukapheresis, although there is a small number of reports in the literature. This procedure could be indicated as supportive care when WBC is over 100,000/mm^3, but it is not always effective. Table 2.1 summarizes all the treatment options discussed.

Table 2.1 Treatment options for CML during pregnancy

	1st trimester	2nd trimester	3rd trimester	Breastfeeding
TKI[a]	No	No	Maybe	No
Hydroxyurea	No	No	No	No
Interferon-alfa	Probably	Yes	Yes	Yes
Leukapheresis	Yes	Yes	Yes	Yes

[a]Even though imatinib is the most studied TKI in pregnancy, yet nilotinib seems to be safe. Other TKIs are not recommended at this time

After the infant is born, the mother can finally restart TKI therapy. However, TKIs are secreted into milk; hence, breastfeeding is contraindicated for women on active treatment. Patients still maintaining major molecular response (MMR) after discontinuation may continue off treatment and can breastfeed. Women on IFN-α can also breastfeed as long as the disease is under good control.

2.3.1.2 Planning Pregnancy in Well-Controlled CML

Family planning is a common concern for younger patients with CP CML. As TKI therapy does not seem to significantly impair fertility, all women of child-bearing age should be advised about contraception while on active treatment because TKI exposure in pregnancy is associated with miscarriage and fetal abnormalities. It is always important to balance the current status of disease and the patient values and preferences, informing about the specific risks of stopping TKI therapy. Traditionally, successful CML treatment depends on good adherence to TKIs maintained lifelong. In recent years though many trials investigated the possibility of TKI therapy discontinuation in selected patients in deep, prolonged molecular remissions [97].

The Euro-Ski trial [99] was a large international, multicenter, prospective study that enrolled over 750 patients with CP CML who had received imatinib, nilotinib, or dasatinib for at least 3 years and had confirmed deep molecular responses (BCR-ABL1 ≤ 0.01% on the International Scale) for at least 1 year. At 24 months after stopping TKI treatment, half of the patients had lost major molecular response (MMR, that is, BCR-ABL1 > 0.1% on the International Scale), most of them in the first 6 months. No serious adverse events were reported and 86% of patients regained MMR after reinitiating TKI therapy.

Based on these data, when a deep molecular response is achieved and sustained, treatment with TKI could be stopped in women planning to become pregnant (Fig. 2.3), either with or without in vitro fertilization [97]. Individualized decisions can be made in patients with good molecular responses, but not as deep or durable enough to meet the criteria for stopping trials. Some groups suggest that TKI cessation before pregnancy could be possible in case of stable MMR for at least 2 years [86, 96, 100]. Given that first-line treatment for CML with dasatinib or nilotinib is able to provide deeper and faster responses compared to imatinib, it is also reasonable to start therapy with a second-generation TKI in women of reproductive age, willing to get pregnant in the near future.

Molecular monitoring by quantitative PCR should be performed every 1 or 2 months after stopping TKI therapy and during pregnancy. Prenatal ob-gyn counseling must take place early. If MMR is lost, treatment with IFN-α may be considered and its dose may be titrated according to tolerance and response. A more conservative approach consists in holding therapy until BCR-ABL levels are over 1%, or at the time of loss of complete cytogenetic response or hematologic response, especially during the first trimester.

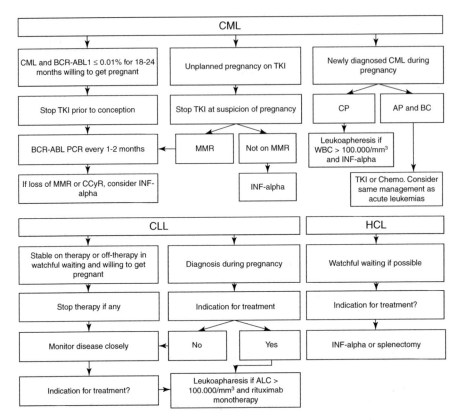

Fig. 2.3 Summary of clinical approach for chronic leukemias. CML chronic myeloid leukemia, TKI tyrosine kinase inhibitor, CP chronic phase, AP accelerated phase, BC blastic crisis, MMR major molecular remission, CCyR complete cytogenetic response, WBC white blood cell count, CLL chronic lymphocytic leukemia, HCL hairy cell leukemia, ALC absolute lymphocyte count

2.3.1.3 Unplanned Pregnancy While on TKI

An unexpected pregnancy may also occur during TKI treatment despite contraception use. In this case, the TKI must be immediately interrupted once the pregnancy is confirmed. If a patient is in MMR, she could rather be observed and closely monitored. If not, IFN-α should be started. An alternative option is the reintroduction of a TKI during the third trimester, particularly in cases of hematologic relapse and intolerance/refractoriness to IFN-α.

2.3.1.4 Pregnant Woman Is Diagnosed with CML

Another possible scenario would be a first diagnosis of CML during pregnancy. For those women in CP with significant leukocytosis (WBC count >100,000/mm³), leukapheresis is a possible option and can be started since the first trimester. In the presence of thrombocytosis (platelet count >500,000/mm³), low-dose aspirin should be started along with prophylactic dose of low-molecular weight heparin for thromboembolism prevention. From the first trimester onward, IFN-α is a good choice, aiming for hematologic response. TKIs may also be considered in selected cases after the period of organogenesis and placental formation.

Managing accelerated or blast phase CML presenting during pregnancy is an even more challenging situation. These patients require early treatment with TKIs, and those with blast crisis usually need induction chemotherapy. Risks and benefits concerning the patient and the fetus should be thoroughly examined with the family. If specific treatment cannot be delayed, pregnancy termination may be discussed with the parents. If diagnosis occurs after week 34–35, a viable option is to consider delivery.

2.3.2 Chronic Lymphocytic Leukemia

Chronic lymphocytic leukemia (CLL) is the most prevalent adult leukemia in the Western world. It is predominantly a disease of the elderly with median age at diagnosis around 60–70 years and with an incidence rate two times higher in men. Only 10–15% of patients are younger than 50 years at diagnosis, and it is estimated that 2% are women of childbearing age [91, 101]; thus, CLL is scarcely ever associated with pregnancy [91, 101]. Only few cases have been reported, all with good outcomes [101]. Even though no guidelines can be outlined in view of the paucity of reports, some considerations can be made. Given its indolent clinical course, CLL treatment can often be withheld until postpartum [91, 101]. Early-stage disease will usually allow a watch-and-wait approach and avoid treatment-related risks to the fetus. Follow up with clinical evaluation, routine blood tests and, in particular cases, ultrasound to evaluate lymph nodes status are mostly sufficient. Therapeutic termination of pregnancy is likely unnecessary. In the urgency to treat, leukapheresis has been successfully used for cytoreduction as a transient measure until partum, after which conventional therapy can be initiated [91].

As a physiological effect of pregnancy, WBC begins to increase in the first trimester, mainly caused by an absolute increase in neutrophils, and peaks during the second and third trimesters, returning to normal ranges within the first week post delivery [101]. Case reports of CLL during pregnancy also reveal an increase in WBC, but this increase is mainly associated with higher absolute lymphocyte count (ALC), followed by a decrease after delivery. ALC sometimes remains above the normal range but lower than the gestational peak, suggesting ALC escalation during pregnancy might be related with pregnancy rather than disease progression [101–104]. Pregnancy hormones may provoke a similar response to that seen in patients initiating treatment for CLL with steroids and B-cell receptor pathway inhibitors, situations in which a transient increment in ALC is observed due to leukocyte redistribution from tissue sites into the circulation [101, 105]. Sex hormones may also have immunomodulatory effects that lead to an increase in immune tolerance during pregnancy, allowing expansion of the monoclonal population of B-lymphocytes. After delivery, the patient's state of immunity returns to its normal, and the monoclonal population decreases in number [102]. Although it has been hypothesized that reproductive factors may affect the risk for lymphoid malignancies and enhance tumor progression, so far the immunological alterations of pregnancy have not been proven to have any relevance on the etiology of CLL [101].

2.3.2.1 Management Considerations

Leukostasis is rarely seen in CLL [101]. Patients usually tolerate ALC as high as 500,000/mm^3 without any symptoms [106]. However, during pregnancy, there are additional potential risks of placental insufficiency, intrauterine growth restriction, and other antenatal complications that need to be considered [101]. In these scenarios, leukapheresis may be used for cytoreduction [106]. Although there is no specific trigger for ALC alone to indicate treatment, some authors have suggested keeping ALC below 100,000/mm^3 in pregnant women [101, 106]. Only one case reported to date applied leukapheresis for CLL during pregnancy [106]. Three sessions were performed, aiming to keep ALC below 100,000/mm^3 [106]. The patient had anemia and thrombocytopenia due to bone marrow infiltration, which did not improve or worsen after leukapheresis [106]. On the other hand, another case whose ALC remained between 100 and 200,000/mm^3 during the entire gestation and who did not receive leukapheresis developed no maternal or fetal complications [107].

Despite the wide range of drugs available nowadays, most CLL patients are candidates to watch-and-wait as initial approach [91, 101] (Fig. 2.3). There is only one case of CLL during pregnancy reported in the literature in which the fetus was exposed to chemotherapy [108]. The patient was on the 3rd month of treatment with chlorambucil and found out a 20-week pregnancy [103]. Chlorambucil was discontinued; no other treatment was required throughout pregnancy; and she gave birth to a healthy baby [107]. Chlorambucil is a category D drug (positive evidence of risk), and exposure to chlorambucil in the first trimester has been associated with congenital abnormalities including renal agenesis, ureteral malformations, and cardiovascular anomalies [33, 101]. Among other drugs used for CLL, fludarabine and cyclophosphamide are also category D. Exposure to cyclophosphamide in the first trimester has been associated with fetal malformation, but it seems to be safe in the second and third trimesters [101].

Rituximab is a category C drug (risk cannot be ruled out); thus, it is not recommended during pregnancy. It crosses the placenta from week 16 onwards, achieving fetal serum levels similar to maternal levels. It can cause neonatal lymphopenia and/or B-cell depletion when administered in the second and third trimesters, which takes up to 6 months to normalize after birth [101]. A review reported 153 pregnancies with known outcomes after maternal exposure to rituximab [118]. Ninety gestations resulted in live births, 22 infants were born prematurely, and few neonatal infections occurred. Only two cases of congenital malformations were observed, with no clear relation to rituximab. These results are also confounded by concomitant use of other medications and severe underlying maternal disease. Even though rituximab appears to have no teratogenic potential, pregnancy should still be avoided for 12 months after last exposure if possible [88].

Ofatumumab and obinutuzumab, other anti-CD20 antibodies, and venetoclax are also category C drugs [101, 105]. Ibrutinib and idelalisib are category D drugs [105]. Lenalidomide is structurally related to thalidomide, a highly teratogenic drug, and is therefore category X, that is, contraindicated in pregnancy [101]. Although so far in the literature no drug treatment to CLL was required during pregnancy, rituximab as a single agent might be the most reasonable choice to temporize treatment if needed [101]. More data on its lower teratogenicity and safety profile are available in comparison with other drugs as it is used in lymphoma and autoimmune diseases [101].

2.3.2.2   Infection Prophylaxis in CLL

Concomitant CLL-related immunosuppression and pregnancy increase the risk for infections [91]. Both mother and fetus are exposed to possible harms [91]. Prophylaxis with inactivated vaccines should be considered [101]. Immunoglobulin G level may be assessed as hypogammaglobulinemia is a common finding in CLL patients, and intravenous immunoglobulin (IVIG) replacement for recurrent or severe infections seems useful and decreases the incidence of bacterial infections in these patients [101].

2.3.2.3   Chronic Lymphocytic Leukemia-Related Cytopenias

Mild anemia and thrombocytopenia are normal findings during pregnancy [106, 109]. However, cytopenias are also common in CLL and can be severe, reflecting either an autoimmune phenomena or marrow failure [106, 107]. Blood transfusion may be required in the setting of marrow infiltration [101, 107]. CLL is also linked to different pathophysiological processes involved in autoimmunity [109]. Usual clinical manifestations are autoimmune hemolytic anemia and immune thrombocytopenia [109]. None of the reported cases had autoimmune manifestations during pregnancy [91, 101–104, 106, 108, 110, 111]. If that happens, corticosteroids may be used [33]. Administration of corticosteroids to any pregnant woman is associated with adverse effects, such as premature rupture of membranes, intrauterine growth restriction, low birth weight, increased infant morbidity, exacerbation of gestational diabetes, and hypertension [109].

2.3.3   Hairy Cell Leukemia

Hairy cell leukemia (HCL) is an uncommon chronic lymphoproliferative disorder with distinctive B-cell immunophenotype, which usually affects the bone marrow, peripheral blood, and spleen. Characteristically, the clinical manifestations are pancytopenia and splenomegaly. It is a rare entity, accounting for only 2% of all leukemias; the median age at diagnosis is around 60 years, and it is more common among men [112]. During pregnancy, it is even more infrequent, but some cases have been reported in the literature over the last decades.

Patients with HCL should receive active treatment only when symptomatic. In general, treatment is indicated if a significant cytopenia is present: hemoglobin <11 g/dL, platelet count <100,000/mm^3 ,or absolute neutrophil count <1000/mm^3. The treatment backbone is based on purine analogs, either cladribine or pentostatin, which provide high response rates and long-term progression-free survival, usually over 10 years [113, 114]. However, using purine analogs during pregnancy is quite concerning, as teratogenic effects have been demonstrated in animal models [115], and the evidence in humans is limited. Other treatment options include monoclonal antibodies (rituximab), interferon-alfa, and splenectomy.

Rituximab has been proven to be effective as monotherapy in HCL, but it has a synergic effect with purine analogs, such as increased complete response rates and minimal residual disease eradication. Chemoimmunotherapy (rituximab + cladribine or pentostatin) is commonly indicated as second-line treatment for relapsed patients, although it may also improve outcomes if used upfront [113, 114].

A single case report described a pregnant woman who presented with HCL in the second trimester and was treated with rituximab and cladribine. She had pancytopenia at diagnosis and received four doses of rituximab in the 26th week of pregnancy with no response. Cladribine was then initiated in week 32, leading to improvement in the blood counts and successful delivery at term. Despite the favorable outcome, more data are necessary to support this approach, and these agents should always be avoided during the first trimester.

Interferon-α was the first effective systemic treatment for HCL. This agent is able to induce remission in most of the cases, although only a partial response is usually achieved. Besides, IFN-α has a slower onset of action and lower durability of remissions compared to purine analogs. It does not inhibit DNA synthesis and is generally safe to use during pregnancy [98]. Two pregnant patients with HCL were treated with IFN-α in a case series and both did not have complications during pregnancy and delivery [116].

Splenectomy is another historical therapy used for HCL. It is not capable of modifying disease biology, though blood counts may considerably improve after the procedure. There are few case reports on splenectomy in the literature, but it appears to be feasible in the second trimester, when the uterus is yet not so enlarged. One case of laparoscopic splenectomy in a pregnant patient with HCL has been reported, showing transitory cytopenia control and good pregnancy outcome [117].

In summary, IFN-α could be considered if HCL requires treatment during pregnancy, given its good efficacy and safety profile [114]. Splenectomy is a possible option in the second trimester (Fig. 2.3). Other medical treatments, including rituximab and cladribine, must be used with caution, weighing risks versus benefits on an individual basis. Often HCL patients will need definitive treatment with purine analogs after delivery.

2.4 Supportive Treatment and Imaging Considerations in Acute and Chronic Leukemias

Blood cell product transfusion should be used as clinically indicated. As for any patient with hematologic malignancies, blood products must be leukocyte-depleted and irradiated. Rh(D) alloimmunization prevention should follow standard guidelines [23].

For patients with non-APL acute leukemias and chronic leukemias without immune cytopenias and no active bleeding, there are no specific guidelines on transfusion triggers for red blood cells and platelets; thus, the decision on providing blood transfusion is to be made on clinical and hematological grounds [118, 119]. We generally recommend keeping hemoglobin levels >7–8 g/dL and platelets counts >20–30,000/mm^3 during pregnancy in the absence of complicating features.

Acute promyelocytic leukemia is a special situation because it is associated with more coagulopathy than other acute leukemias. Special awareness should be paid to not misdiagnose APL for HELLP syndrome. It is mandatory to assess prothrombin time (PT), partial thromboplastin time (PTT), fibrinogen, and platelets to make the distinction. In APL, all coagulation alterations should be corrected immediately. Fibrinogen concentrate should be given to achieve fibrinogen levels of at least 150 mg/dL [25]. If fibrinogen concentrate is not available, cryoprecipitate could be used. If PT and PTT are still abnormal after correction of fibrinogen levels, fresh frozen plasma should be administered. Platelets should be kept above 50,000/mm^3 [25].

Growth factor support with GCSF can be used during pregnancy if clinically indicated [4, 32, 120]. Other supportive drugs (e.g., infection prophylaxis) will be described in detail in Chaps. 7 and 8.

Even though computed-tomography (CT) and positron emission tomography–computed tomography (PET-CT) scans are to be avoided during pregnancy, risks and benefits need to be weighed. MRI should not be performed in the first trimester but can be performed in the second and third trimesters with gadolinium if strongly indicated [35].

2.5　Delivery Considerations

Chemotherapy should be stopped 3–4 weeks before delivery to allow hematologic recovery of mother and fetus. Transfusion of blood components should be used to achieve safe platelets thresholds at delivery. In line with current guidelines, platelet count should be >50,000/mm^3 before delivery and >70–80,000/mm^3 for epidural or spinal anesthesia [23, 119]. Details about types of delivery in women with leukemia are discussed in Chap. 6.

2.6　Postpartum Considerations

Consolidation therapy, including hematopoietic stem cell transplant (HSCT) if indicated, should be pursued as soon as possible after recovery from delivery. After an uncomplicated cesarean delivery, the recommendation is to wait 1 week [7]. Women must be advised to avoid a new pregnancy for 2–3 years following the end of acute leukemia treatment [4, 7] due to the risk of recurrence. For chronic leukemias, a subsequent pregnancy should be carefully planned, taking the disease control status and current therapy into consideration. It is important to initiate deep venous thrombosis (DVT) prophylaxis if possible, given the combined risk for DVT associated with postpartum and malignancy. Breastfeeding recommendations are discussed in detail in Chap. 10.

References

1. Pavlidis NA. Coexistence of pregnancy and malignancy. Oncologist. 2002;7(4):279–87.
2. Calsteren K van, Heyns L, Smet FD, Eycken LV, Gziri MM, Gemert WV, et al. Cancer during pregnancy: an analysis of 215 patients emphasizing the obstetrical and the neonatal outcomes. 689 [Internet]. 2010. [cited 2019 Oct 8]; Available from: https://repository.ubn.ru.nl/handle/2066/88224
3. Chelghoum Y, Vey N, Raffoux E, Huguet F, Pigneux A, Witz B, et al. Acute leukemia during pregnancy: a report on 37 patients and a review of the literature. Cancer. 2005;104(1):110–7.
4. Brenner B, Avivi I, Lishner M. Haematological cancers in pregnancy. Lancet. 2012;379(9815):580–7.
5. Osada S, Horibe K, Oiwa K, Yoshida J, Iwamura H, Matsuoka H, et al. A case of infantile acute monocytic leukemia caused by vertical transmission of the mother's leukemic cells. Cancer. 1990;65(5):1146–9.
6. Greenlund LJS, Letendre L, Tefferi A. Acute leukemia during pregnancy: a single institutional experience with 17 cases. Leuk Lymphoma. 2001;41(5–6):571–7.
7. Thomas, X. Acute myeloid leukemia in the pregnant patient. Eur J Haematol. Accepted Author Manuscript. 2015. https://doi.org/10.1111/ejh.12535.
8. Requena A, Velasco JG, Pinilla J, Gonzalez-Gonzalez A. Acute leukemia during pregnancy: obstetric management and perinatal outcome of two cases. Eur J Obstet Gynecol Reprod Biol. 1995;63(2):139–41.

9. Cardonick E, Iacobucci A. Use of chemotherapy during human pregnancy. Lancet Oncol. 2004;5(5):283–91.
10. van Hasselt JGC, van Calsteren K, Heyns L, Han S, Mhallem Gziri M, Schellens JHM, et al. Optimizing anticancer drug treatment in pregnant cancer patients: pharmacokinetic analysis of gestation-induced changes for doxorubicin, epirubicin, docetaxel and paclitaxel. Ann Oncol. 2014;25(10):2059–65.
11. Avilés A, Neri N, Nambo M-J. Hematological malignancies and pregnancy: treat or no treat during first trimester. Int J Cancer. 2012;131(11):2678–83.
12. Farhadfar N, Cerquozzi S, Hessenauer MR, Litzow MR, Hogan WJ, Letendre L, et al. Acute leukemia in pregnancy: a single institution experience with 23 patients. Leuk Lymphoma. 2017;58(5):1052–60.
13. Molkenboer JF, Vos AH, Schouten HC, Vos MC. Acute lymphoblastic leukaemia in pregnancy. Neth J Med. 2005;63(9):361–3.
14. Zaidi A, Johnson L-M, Church CL, Gomez-Garcia WC, Popescu MI, Margolin JF, et al. Management of concurrent pregnancy and acute lymphoblastic malignancy in teenaged patients: two illustrative cases and review of the literature. J Adolesc Young Adult Oncol. 2014;3(4):160–75.
15. Avilés A, Neri N. Hematological malignancies and pregnancy: a final report of 84 children who received chemotherapy in utero. Clin Lymphoma. 2001;2(3):173–7.
16. Avilés A, Díaz-Maqueo JC, Talavera A, Guzmán R, García EL. Growth and development of children of mothers treated with chemotherapy during pregnancy: current status of 43 children. Am J Hematol. 1991;36(4):243–8.
17. Queisser-Luft A, Stolz G, Wiesel A, Schlaefer K, Spranger J. Malformations in newborn: results based on 30,940 infants and fetuses from the Mainz congenital birth defect monitoring system (1990-1998). Arch Gynecol Obstet. 2002;266(3):163–7.
18. Doll DC, Ringenberg QS, Yarbro JW. Management of cancer during pregnancy. Arch Intern Med. 1988;148(9):2058–64.
19. Weisz B, Meirow D, Schiff E, Lishner M. Impact and treatment of cancer during pregnancy. Expert Rev Anticancer Ther. 2004;4(5):889–902.
20. Selig BP, Furr JR, Huey RW, Moran C, Alluri VN, Medders GR, et al. Cancer chemotherapeutic agents as human teratogens. Birt Defects Res A Clin Mol Teratol. 2012;94(8):626–50.
21. Ticku J, Oberoi S, Friend S, Busowski J, Langenstroer M, Baidas S. Acute lymphoblastic leukemia in pregnancy: a case report with literature review. Ther Adv Hematol. 2013;4(5):313–9.
22. Vlijm-Kievit A, Jorna NG, Moll E, Pajkrt E, Pals ST, Middeldorp S, et al. Acute lymphoblastic leukemia during the third trimester of pregnancy. Leuk Lymphoma. 2018;59(5):1274–6.
23. Ali S, Jones GL, Culligan DJ, Marsden PJ, Russell N, Embleton ND, et al. Guidelines for the diagnosis and management of acute myeloid leukaemia in pregnancy. Br J Haematol. 2015;170(4):487–95.
24. Cuttner J, Holland JF, Norton L, Ambinder E, Button G, Meyer RJ. Therapeutic leukapheresis for hyperleukocytosis in acute myelocytic leukemia. Med Pediatr Oncol. 1983;11(2):76–8.
25. NCCN Clinical Practice Guidelines in Oncology (NCCN Guidelines) – Acute myeloid leukemia. Version 2.2019 — March 8, 2019.
26. Reynoso EE, Shepherd FA, Messner HA, Farquharson HA, Garvey MB, Baker MA. Acute leukemia during pregnancy: the Toronto Leukemia Study Group experience with long-term follow-up of children exposed in utero to chemotherapeutic agents. J Clin Oncol Off J Am Soc Clin Oncol. 1987;5(7):1098–106.
27. Caligiuri MA, Mayer RJ. Pregnancy and leukemia. Semin Oncol. 1989;16(5):388–96.
28. Horowitz NA, Henig I, Henig O, Benyamini N, Vidal L, Avivi I. Acute myeloid leukemia during pregnancy: a systematic review and meta-analysis. Leuk Lymphoma. 2018;59(3):610–6.
29. Siu BL, Alonzo MR, Vargo TA, Fenrich AL. Transient dilated cardiomyopathy in a newborn exposed to idarubicin and all-trans-retinoic acid (ATRA) early in the second trimester of pregnancy. Int J Gynecol Cancer. 2002;12(4):399–402.

30. Maruyama S, Sato Y, Moriuchi K, Kanbayashi S, Ri Y, Taga A, et al. Fetal death following idarubicin treatment for acute promyelocytic leukemia in pregnancy—a case report. Eur J Obstet Gynecol Reprod Biol. 2017;218:140.
31. Achtari C, Hohlfeld P. Cardiotoxic transplacental effect of idarubicin administered during the second trimester of pregnancy. Am J Obstet Gynecol. 2000;183(2):511–2.
32. Azim HA Jr, Pavlidis N, Peccatori FA. Treatment of the pregnant mother with cancer: a systematic review on the use of cytotoxic, endocrine, targeted agents and immunotherapy during pregnancy. Part II: hematological tumors. Cancer Treat Rev. 2010;36(2):110–21.
33. Shapira T, Pereg D, Lishner M. How I treat acute and chronic leukemia in pregnancy. Blood Rev. 2008;22(5):247–59.
34. Lavi N, Horowitz NA, Brenner B. An update on the management of hematologic malignancies in pregnancy. Womens Health. 2014;10(3):255–66.
35. Peccatori FA, Azim HA Jr, Orecchia R, Hoekstra HJ, Pavlidis N, Kesic V, et al. Cancer, pregnancy and fertility: ESMO clinical practice guidelines for diagnosis, treatment and follow-up. Ann Oncol. 2013;24(suppl_6):vi160–70.
36. Germann N, Goffinet F, Goldwasser F. Anthracyclines during pregnancy: embryo–fetal outcome in 160 patients. Ann Oncol. 2004;15(1):146–50.
37. Yates J, Glidewell O, Wiernik P, Cooper MR, Steinberg D, Dosik H, et al. Cytosine arabinoside with daunorubicin or adriamycin for therapy of acute myelocytic leukemia: a CALGB study. Blood. 1982;60(2):454–62.
38. Doxorubicin versus Idarubicin with overall survival in adult acute myeloid leukemia patients| Abstract [Internet]. [cited 2019 Oct 17]. Available from: https://www.alliedacademies.org/proceedings/doxorubicin-versus-idarubicin-with-overall-survival-in-adult-acute-myeloid-leukemia-patients-1462.html
39. Wagner VM, Hill JS, Weaver D, Baehner RL. Congenital abnormalities in baby born to cytarabine treated mother. Lancet Lond Engl. 1980;2(8185):98–9.
40. Schafer AI. Teratogenic effects of antileukemic chemotherapy. Arch Intern Med. 1981;141(4):514–5.
41. Artlich A, Möller J, Kruse K, Gortner L, Tschakaloff A, Schwinger E. Teratogenic effects in a case of maternal treatment for acute myelocytic leukaemia—neonatal and infantile course. Eur J Pediatr. 1994;153(7):488–91.
42. Fernandez HF, Sun Z, Yao X, Litzow MR, Luger SM, Paietta EM, et al. Anthracycline dose intensification in acute myeloid leukemia. N Engl J Med. 2009;361(13):1249–59.
43. Fracchiolla NS, Sciumè M, Dambrosi F, Guidotti F, Ossola MW, Chidini G, et al. Acute myeloid leukemia and pregnancy: clinical experience from a single center and a review of the literature. BMC Cancer. 2017;17(1):442.
44. Sanz MA, Grimwade D, Tallman MS, Lowenberg B, Fenaux P, Estey EH, et al. Management of acute promyelocytic leukemia: recommendations from an expert panel on behalf of the European LeukemiaNet. Blood. 2009;113(9):1875–91.
45. Lammer EJ, Chen DT, Hoar RM, Agnish ND, Benke PJ, Braun JT, et al. Retinoic acid embryopathy. N Engl J Med. 1985;313(14):837–41.
46. Yang D, Hladnik L. Treatment of acute promyelocytic leukemia during pregnancy. Pharmacotherapy. 2009;29(6):709–24.
47. Valappil S, Kurkar M, Howell R. Outcome of pregnancy in women treated with all-trans retinoic acid; a case report and review of literature. Hematol Amst Neth. 2007;12(5):415–8.
48. Fadilah SAW, Hatta AZ, Keng CS, Jamil MA, Singh S. Successful treatment of acute promyelocytic leukemia in pregnancy with all-trans retinoic acid. Leukemia. 2001;15(10):1665.
49. Verma V, Giri S, Manandhar S, Pathak R, Bhatt VR. Acute promyelocytic leukemia during pregnancy: a systematic analysis of outcome. Leuk Lymphoma. 2016;57(3):616–22.
50. Rizack T, Mega A, Legare R, Castillo J. Management of hematological malignancies during pregnancy. Am J Hematol. 2009;84(12):830–41.

51. For the European APL group, Fenaux P, Chevret S, Guerci A, Fegueux N, Dombret H, et al. Long-term follow-up confirms the benefit of all-trans retinoic acid in acute promyelocytic leukemia. Leukemia. 2000;14(8):1371–7.
52. Stahl M, Tallman MS. Differentiation syndrome in acute promyelocytic leukaemia. Br J Haematol. 2019;187(2):157–62.
53. Tallman MS, Andersen JW, Schiffer CA, Appelbaum FR, Feusner JH, Ogden A, et al. All-trans-retinoic acid in acute promyelocytic leukemia. N Engl J Med. 1997;337(15):1021–8.
54. Fenaux P, Chastang C, Chevret S, Sanz M, Dombret H, Archimbaud E, et al. A randomized comparison of all transretinoic acid (ATRA) followed by chemotherapy and ATRA plus chemotherapy and the role of maintenance therapy in newly diagnosed acute promyelocytic leukemia. The European APL Group. Blood. 1999;94(4):1192–200.
55. Culligan DJ, Merriman L, Kell J, Parker J, Jovanovic JV, Smith N, et al. The Management of acute promyelocytic leukemia presenting during pregnancy. Clin Leuk. 2007;1(3):183–91.
56. Sanz MA, Montesinos P, Casale MF, Díaz-Mediavilla J, Jiménez S, Fernández I, et al. Maternal and fetal outcomes in pregnant women with acute promyelocytic leukemia. Ann Hematol. 2015;94(8):1357–61.
57. Adès L, Sanz MA, Chevret S, Montesinos P, Chevallier P, Raffoux E, et al. Treatment of newly diagnosed acute promyelocytic leukemia (APL): a comparison of French-Belgian-Swiss and PETHEMA results. Blood. 2008;111(3):1078–84.
58. Nellessen CM, Janzen V, Mayer K, Giovannini G, Gembruch U, Brossart P, et al. Successful treatment of acute promyelocytic leukemia in pregnancy with single-agent all-trans retinoic acid. Arch Gynecol Obstet. 2018;297(2):281–4.
59. Bottsford-Miller J, Haeri S, Baker AM, Boles J, Brown M. B cell acute lymphocytic leukemia in pregnancy. Arch Gynecol Obstet. 2011;284(2):303–6.
60. Matsouka C, Marinopoulos S, Barbaroussi D, Antsaklis A. Acute lymphoblastic leukemia during gestation. Med Oncol. 2008;25(2):190–3.
61. Nakajima Y, Hattori Y, Ito S, Ohshima R, Kuwabara H, Machida S, et al. Acute leukemia during pregnancy: an investigative survey of the past 11 years. Int J Lab Hematol. 2015;37(2):174–80.
62. Gonçalves R, Meel R. A rare case of massive hepatosplenomegaly due to acute lymphoblastic leukaemia in pregnancy. SAM J South Afr Med J. 2017;107(5):402–4.
63. Ataergin, S., Kanat, O., Arpaci, F. and Ozet, A. A rare occurrence of diffuse lymphoblastic lymphoma in pregnancy. Am. J. Hematol., 2007;82:173–174. https://doi.org/10.1002/ajh.20681.
64. Tewari K, Cappuccini F, Rosen RB, Rosenthal J, Asrat T, Kohler MF. Relapse of acute lymphoblastic leukemia in pregnancy: survival following chemoirradiation and autologous transfer of interleukin-2-activated stem cells. Gynecol Oncol. 1999;74(1):143–6.
65. Brincker H, Christensen BE, Cold S. Two pregnancy-associated late relapses in acute lymphoblastic leukemia. Haematologica. 1989;74(3):289–91.
66. Camera A, Campanile M, Catalano D, Mattace AR, Rotoli B. Relapse of acute lymphoblastic leukemia during pregnancy. Eur J Gynaecol Oncol. 1996;17(4):303–5.
67. Mainor CB, Duffy AP, Atkins KL, Kimball AS, Baer MR. Treatment of Philadelphia chromosome-positive acute lymphoblastic leukemia in pregnancy. J Oncol Pharm Pract. 2016;22(2):374–7.
68. Erkut N, Akidan O, Batur DS, Karabacak V, Sonmez M. Comparison between hyper-CVAD and PETHEMA ALL-93 in adult acute lymphoblastic leukemia: a single-center study. Chemotherapy. 2018;63(4):207–13.
69. Sas V, Moisoiu V, Teodorescu P, Tranca S, Pop L, Iluta S, et al. Approach to the adult acute lymphoblastic leukemia patient. J Clin Med. 2019;8(8):1175.
70. Chalandon Y, Thomas X, Hayette S, Cayuela J-M, Abbal C, Huguet F, et al. Randomized study of reduced-intensity chemotherapy combined with imatinib in adults with Ph-positive acute lymphoblastic leukemia. Blood. 2015;125(24):3711–9.

71. Saleh AJM, Alhejazi A, Ahmed SO, Al Mohareb F, AlSharif F, AlZahrani H, et al. Leukemia during pregnancy: long term follow up of 32 cases from a single institution. Hematol Oncol Stem Cell Ther. 2014;7(2):63–8.
72. Khandaker S, Munshi S. A rare case of acute lymphoblastic leukaemia in pregnancy-unique maternal-fetal challenges. J Clin Diagn Res JCDR. 2014;8(10):OD10.
73. Ali R, Ozkalemkas F, Kimya Y, Koksal N, Ozkan H, Ozkocaman V, et al. Acute leukemia and pregnancy. Leuk Res. 2009;33(3):e26–8.
74. Mahmoud HK, Samra MA, Fathy GM. Hematologic malignancies during pregnancy: a review. J Adv Res. 2016;7(4):589–96.
75. Esin S, Tarim E, Abali H, Kardes O, Kocer EN, Alkan O. Management of precursor B-lymphoblastic lymphoma/leukaemia of thoracic spine in a pregnancy presenting with acute paraplegia. Lancet Oncol. 2012;5:283–91.
76. Kekre N, Connors JM. Venous thromboembolism incidence in hematologic malignancies. Blood Rev. 2019;33:24–32.
77. Piatkowska-Jakubas B, Krawczyk-Kuliś M, Giebel S, Adamczyk-Cioch M, Czyz A, Lech ME, et al. Use of L-asparaginase in acute lymphoblastic leukemia: recommendations of the Polish Adult Leukemia Group. Pol Arch Med Wewn. 2008;118(11):664–9.
78. Goyal G, Bhatt VR. L-asparaginase and venous thromboembolism in acute lymphocytic leukemia. Future Oncol. 2015;11(17):2459–70.
79. Hochhaus A, Saussele S, Rosti G, Mahon F-X, Janssen JJ, Hjorth-Hansen H, et al. Chronic myeloid leukaemia: ESMO clinical practice guidelines for diagnosis, treatment and follow-up. Ann Oncol. 2017;28(suppl_4):iv41–51.
80. Balsat M, Etienne M, Elhamri M, Hayette S, Salles G, Thomas X. Successful pregnancies in patients with BCR-ABL-positive leukemias treated with interferon-alpha therapy during the tyrosine kinase inhibitors era. Eur J Haematol. 2018;101(6):774–80.
81. Yilmaz M, Kantarjian H, Ravandi-Kashani F, Short NJ, Jabbour E. Philadelphia chromosome-positive acute lymphoblastic leukemia in adults: current treatments and future perspectives. Clin Adv Hematol Oncol. 2018;16(3):216–23.
82. Pye SM, Cortes J, Ault P, Hatfield A, Kantarjian H, Pilot R, et al. The effects of imatinib on pregnancy outcome. Blood. 2008;111(12):5505–8.
83. Cortes JE, Abruzzese E, Chelysheva E, Guha M, Wallis N, Apperley JF. The impact of dasatinib on pregnancy outcomes. Am J Hematol. 2015;90(12):1111–5.
84. Berveiller P, Andreoli A, Mir O, Anselem O, Delezoide A-L, Sauvageon H, et al. A dramatic fetal outcome following transplacental transfer of dasatinib. Anti-Cancer Drugs. 2012;23(7):754–7.
85. Barkoulas T, Hall PD. Experience with dasatinib and nilotinib use in pregnancy. J Oncol Pharm Pract. 2018;24(2):121–8.
86. Abruzzese E, Trawinska MM, de Fabritiis P, Baccarani M. Management of pregnant chronic myeloid leukemia patients. Expert Rev Hematol. 2016;9(8):781–91.
87. Ahmad H, Mehta NJ, Lamoste VM, Lamoste TJ, Chapnick EK, Lutwick LI, et al. Pneumocystis carinii pneumonia in pregnancy. Chest. 2001;120(2):666–71.
88. Daver N, Nazha A, Kantarjian HM, Haltom R, Ravandi F. Treatment of hairy cell leukemia during pregnancy: are purine analogues and rituximab viable therapeutic options. Clin Lymphoma Myeloma Leuk. 2013;13(1):86.
89. Chen Y, Wang H, Kantarjian H, Cortes J. Trends in chronic myeloid leukemia incidence and survival in the United States from 1975 to 2009. Leuk Lymphoma. 2013;54(7):1411–7.
90. SEER lifetime risk (percent) of being diagnosed with cancer by site and race/ethnicity: both sexes, 18 SEER areas, 2012-2014 (Table 1.15) National Cancer Institute, Bethesda, MD. [Internet]. [cited 2019 Dec 27]. Available from: https://seer.cancer.gov/csr/1975_2014/results_merged/topic_lifetime_risk.pdf.
91. Winckler P, Vanazzi A, Bozzo M, Scarfone G, Peccatori FA. Chronic lymphocytic leukaemia during pregnancy: management and thoughts. Ecancermedicalscience. 2015;9:592.

92. Jabbour E, Kantarjian H. Chronic myeloid leukemia: 2018 update on diagnosis, therapy and monitoring. Am J Hematol. 2018;93(3):442–59.
93. Law AD, Dong Hwan Kim D, Lipton JH. Pregnancy: part of life in chronic myelogenous leukemia. Leuk Lymphoma. 2017;58(2):280–7.
94. NCCN Clinical Practice Guidelines in Oncology (NCCN Guidelines) – Chronic myeloid leukemia. Version 2.2020 – September 25,2019.
95. Baccarani M, Deininger MW, Rosti G, Hochhaus A, Soverini S, Apperley JF, et al. European LeukemiaNet recommendations for the management of chronic myeloid leukemia: 2013. Blood J Am Soc Hematol. 2013;122(6):872–84.
96. Palani R, Milojkovic D, Apperley JF. Managing pregnancy in chronic myeloid leukemia. In: Chronic myeloid leukemia. Cham, Switzerland: Springer; 2016;161–75.
97. Berman E, Druker BJ, Burwick R. Chronic Myelogenous leukemia: pregnancy in the era of stopping tyrosine kinase inhibitor therapy. J Clin Oncol Off J Am Soc Clin Oncol. 2018;36(12):1250.
98. Brojeni PY, Matok I, Bournissen FG, Koren G. A systematic review of the fetal safety of interferon alpha. Reprod Toxicol. 2012;33(3):265–8.
99. Saussele S, Richter J, Guilhot J, Gruber FX, Hjorth-Hansen H, Almeida A, et al. Discontinuation of tyrosine kinase inhibitor therapy in chronic myeloid leukaemia (EURO-SKI): a prespecified interim analysis of a prospective, multicentre, non-randomised, trial. Lancet Oncol. 2018;19(6):747–57.
100. Marlise R. Luskin. Chronic myeloid leukemia and pregnancy: patient and partner perspectives, Expert Review of Hematology, Switzerland. 2018:11(8);597–599. https://doi.org/1 0.1080/17474086.2018.1500889.
101. Hamad N, Kliman D, Best OG, Caramins M, Hertzberg M, Lindeman R, et al. Chronic lymphocytic leukaemia, monoclonal B-lymphocytosis and pregnancy: five cases, a literature review and discussion of management. Br J Haematol. 2015;168(3):350–60.
102. Welsh TM, Thompson J, Lim S. Chronic lymphocytic leukemia in pregnancy. Leukemia. 2000;14(6):1155.
103. Gürman G. Pregnancy and successful labor in the course of chronic lymphocytic leukemia. Am J Hematol. 2002;71(3):208–10.
104. Chrisomalis L, Baxi LV, Heller D. Chronic lymphocytic leukemia in pregnancy. Am J Obstet Gynecol. 1996;175(5):1381–2.
105. Burger JA, O'Brien S. Evolution of CLL treatment—from chemoimmunotherapy to targeted and individualized therapy. Nat Rev Clin Oncol. 2018;15(8):510.
106. Tahmasebi F, Hussain K, Smart G, Gupta M, Hossain U. Successful pregnancy in the context of previously undiagnosed chronic lymphocytic leukaemia: a case report and literature review. Obstet Med. 2017;10(4):189–91.
107. Ali R, Özkalemkaş F, Özkocaman V, Bülbül-Başkan E, Özçelik T, Ozan Ü, et al. Successful labor in the course of chronic lymphocytic leukemia (CLL) and management of CLL during pregnancy with leukapheresis. Ann Hematol. 2004;83(1):61–3.
108. Ali R, Ozkalemkas F, Kimya Y, Koksal N, Ozkocaman V, Yorulmaz H, et al. Pregnancy in chronic lymphocytic leukemia: experience with fetal exposure to chlorambucil. Leuk Res. 2009;33(4):567–9.
109. Jønsson V, Bock JE, Hilden J, Houlston RS, Wiik A. The influence of pregnancy on the development of autoimmunity in chronic lymphocytic leukemia. Leuk Lymphoma. 2006;47(8):1481–7.
110. Ali R, Özkalemkaş F, Özkocaman V, Özçelik T, Ozan Ü, Kimya Y, et al. Successful pregnancy and delivery in a patient with chronic myelogenous leukemia (CML), and management of CML with leukapheresis during pregnancy: a case report and review of the literature. Jpn J Clin Oncol. 2004;34(4):215–7.
111. Maxwell C, Grady R, Crump M. Chronic lymphocytic leukaemia in pregnancy: a case report and literature review. Obstet Med. 2009;2(4):168–9.

112. Kreitman RJ. Hairy cell leukemia: present and future directions. Leuk Lymphoma. 2019;60(12):2869–2879.
113. Grever MR, Abdel-Wahab O, Andritsos LA, Banerji V, Barrientos J, Blachly JS, et al. Consensus guidelines for the diagnosis and management of patients with classic hairy cell leukemia. Blood J Am Soc Hematol. 2017;129(5):553–60.
114. Maitre E, Cornet E, Troussard X. Hairy cell leukemia: 2020 update on diagnosis, risk stratification, and treatment. Am J Hematol. 2019;94:1413.
115. Lau C, Narotsky MG, Lui D, Best D, Setzer RW, Mann PC, et al. Exposure-disease continuum for 2-chloro-2′-deoxyadenosine (2-CdA), a prototype teratogen: induction of lumbar hernia in the rat and species comparison for the teratogenic responses. Teratology. 2002;66(1):6–18.
116. Baer MR, Ozer H, Foon KA. Interferon-α therapy during pregnancy in chronic myelogenous leukaemia and hairy cell leukaemia. Br J Haematol. 1992;81(2):167–9.
117. Adeniji BA, Fallas M, Incerpi M, Hamburg S, Katz R, Ogunyemi D. Laparoscopic splenectomy for hairy cell leukemia in pregnancy. Case Rep Med. 2010;2010:136823.
118. Gernsheimer T, James AH, Stasi R. How I treat thrombocytopenia in pregnancy. Blood. 2013;121(1):38–47.
119. ACOG Practice Bulletin No. 207: thrombocytopenia in pregnancy. Obstet Gynecol. 2019;133(3):e181–93.
120. Dale DC, Cottle TE, Fier CJ, Bolyard AA, Bonilla MA, Boxer LA, et al. Severe chronic neutropenia: treatment and follow-up of patients in the Severe Chronic Neutropenia International Registry. Am J Hematol. 2003;72(2):82–93.

Chapter 3
Chemotherapy Protocols for Leukemia During Pregnancy

Kaléu Mormino Otoni, Karla Bruna Nogueira Torres Mormino, Ranieri Sales de Souza Santos, and Aline Rebeca de Sousa Magalhães

3.1 Introduction

During the gestational period, frequent monitoring of the woman's health in prenatal consultations, recurrent use of ultrasound exams, in addition to greater sensitivity, and precaution of the pregnant woman with her own body and health can support the diagnosis of neoplasms in different stages of development [1].

The diagnosis of leukemia brings suffering to the pregnant woman and generates emotional conflicts, in addition to great distress of health professionals (uneasiness with the therapeutic conduct and prognosis of the patient and the fetus) in the monitoring of the related patient. Such concern lies in the reserved prognosis, especially in the limitation of treatment options, especially if the pregnant woman is in the first trimester [2].

With regard specifically to antineoplastic treatment, it is necessary to measure the maternal risk/benefit and mainly the consequences for the fetus, as well as the results for the woman's reproductive future. Gestational age, stage, and aggressiveness of the neoplasia are fundamental in the interferences of the whole treatment. In view of this, a complete multidisciplinary team (composed of, for example, obstetrician, oncologist, psychologist, and nurse) is always a priority and a primary factor, as well as contributing to the decision of the respective mother; we also have to emphasize the presence of the pharmaceutical professional [3].

In general, there are still controversies about the type of conduct, whether or not to perform surgical interventions, termination of pregnancy, use of chemotherapy or radiation therapy, and even a ban on possible future pregnancies—although the

K. M. Otoni (✉)
Pronutrir Nutritional Support and Chemotherapy Ltda, Fortaleza, Ceará, Brazil

K. B. N. T. Mormino · R. S. de Souza Santos · A. R. de Sousa Magalhães
Catholic University Center of Quixadá, Quixadá, Ceará, Brazil

© Springer Nature Switzerland AG 2021
C. W. P. Schmidt, K. M. Otoni (eds.), *Chemotherapy and Pharmacology for Leukemia in Pregnancy*, https://doi.org/10.1007/978-3-030-54058-6_3

Table 3.1 Gestational age and potential risks to the fetus

Gestational age	Potential risks to the fetus
Preimplantation	About 1.5% abortion (studies with animals) 50% abortion (studies with animals)
1–8 weeks	Mental retardation, microcephaly, and malformations in multiple organs
8–15 weeks	Mental retardation; microcephaly; and bone, ocular, and genital malformations
15–25 weeks	Growth restriction, lower risk of structural malformations, possible risk of microcephaly, and mental retardation
Above 30 weeks	Increased risk of radio-induced cancer and intrauterine growth restriction

Source: Adapted from Freitas (2011)

specificity and sensitivity of the techniques, antineoplastic drugs, and the different types of neoplasia are quite advanced in the current scientific world [4].

According to Table 3.1, it is clear that, over the weeks, the potential risk to the fetus increases. Thus, it is important to know the type of leukemia, the gestational age, the stage, and the aggressiveness of the cancer, so that the correct and appropriate treatment can be done.

However, the delay in starting treatment has severe consequences for both mother and fetus. Leukemia in pregnancy brings with it an increased risk of miscarriage, restriction of fetal growth, and perinatal mortality. Especially for fetal abortion, the causes are in the development of maternal anemia, disseminated intravascular coagulation and changes in blood flow, and in the exchange of nutrients and oxygen supply through the intervillous placental spaces by leukemic cells [5].

The teratogenic risk associated with cancer treatment seems to be lower than that reported in a study with animals, since the doses usually applied in humans are lower than the minimum teratogenic dose applied to animals. However, exposure in the first trimester to chemotherapy results in an increased risk of 10–20% of serious malformations. This risk, however, can be reduced when the chemotherapy intervention is a single agent, when possible, compared with combined chemotherapies [5].

In this chapter, we will present the chemotherapy protocols used in pregnant women with leukemia, emphasizing acute myeloid leukemia (AML), chronic myeloid leukemia (CML), and acute lymphocytic leukemia (ALL).

3.2 Acute Leukemias

Although leukemia is uncommon during pregnancy (representing approximately one case for every 75,000 pregnant women and one case for every 100,000 pregnant women), acute leukemias are responsible for most of these cases. Acute lymphoid leukemia (ALL) accounts for about one-third of cases and acute myeloid leukemia (AML) in two-thirds of cases [5].

Acute leukemias include AML, ALL, and acute promyelocytic leukemia (APL). Therefore, all of them are configured as medical emergencies and if the appropriate and rapid treatment is not undertaken, patients can suffer from bleeding, infections, or organ dysfunctions within days to weeks until death [6].

3.2.1 Acute Myeloid Leukemia (AML)

Acute leukemias result in a malignant transformation of primitive hematopoietic cells, followed by clonal proliferation and, consequently, an increase in these transformed cells. Acute Myeloid Leukemia (AML) characteristically undergoes a maturation cell arrest in the blast or promotion phase, leading to a decrease in normal elements in peripheral blood. The cells exhibit specified myeloid markers, including Auer rods, cytochemical alteration, and applied surface antigens [7].

The kickoff that determines neoplastic proliferation is still unknown; however, it is the result of somatic mutation that occurs in the stem cell, thus compromising myeloid maturity [8]. The incidence of AML by age is 3.6 new cases per 100,000 inhabitants per year, with a median age at diagnosis of 66 years [9]. Therefore, the identification of disease in its early stage is a key factor for the treatment and prognosis.

According to the World Health Organization (WHO), there is a classification for acute myeloblastic leukemia that causes cytogenetic or molecular cytogenetic abnormalities, subdividing them into genetic-clinical-pathological entities [10], as shown in Table 3.2.

The treatment of AML requires initial chemotherapy of remission inducing, in order to achieve complete remission of the disease and consequent restoration of normal blood cells. This phase is continued by post-remission therapy to eradicate minimal residual disease (MRD). After that, two to four "consolidation" courses with or without prolonged "maintenance" treatment. The cure for AML still occurs in a minority of patients who undergo chemotherapy protocols and, in cases of intermediate or unfavorable prognosis, despite the high potential for morbidity, the results of the allogeneic hematopoietic stem cell transplantation (allo-HSCT) or autologous (auto-HSCT) are better than those obtained with standard chemotherapy.

Therefore, the chemotherapy protocols used for AML in pregnant women can be those described in Table 3.3.

When pregnancy is considered recent (in very early stages to think about the possibility of inducing labor), standard treatment protocols that indicate the use of combined chemotherapy are followed: daunorubicin with cytarabine—this is used in the UK. Other international regimes follow the standardization of anthracycline use. It is worth mentioning that there are no records that consider a regime more recommended than another in this situation. However, there are also no records that support an increase in the dose of daunorubicin (90 mg/m^2 D1, D3, D5). Adjusting the

Table 3.2 Classification of AML (WHO)

AML with recurrent genetic abnormalities	AML with t (8,21) (q22; q22); AML 1 / ETO AML with inv (16) (p13; q22); or t (16; 16) (p13; q22); CBFBeta/MYH11 Acute promyelocytic leukemia with t (15; 17) (q22; q12); PML/RARAlfa—AML with 11q23 anomaly; rearrangements MLL/XX
AML with multi-lineage dysplasia	AML without previous myelodysplastic syndrome (MDS) AML after MDS
AML and MDS associated with therapy	AML after alkylating therapy AML after topoisomerase inhibitor Other types
AML not classifiable in the above groups	AML with minimal differentiation (FAB M0) AML without maturation (FAB M1) Matured AML (FAB M2) Acute promyelocytic leukemia (FAB M3) and Variant (FAB M3v) Acute myelomonocytic leukemia (FAB M4) Acute myelomonocytic leukemia with eosinophilia (FAB M4Eo) Acute monoblastic leukemia (FAB M5a) Acute monocytic leukemia (FAB M5b) Acute erythroid leukemia (FAB M6) Acute megacarioblastic leukemia (FAB M7) Acute basophilic leukemia (Baseline FAB M2) Acute panmyelosis with myelofibrosis
Myeloid sarcoma	Myeloid proliferations related to Down syndrome »» Plasmacytoid blast dendritic cell neoplasm
Acute leukemias of ambiguous lineage	Acute undifferentiated leukemia Acute leukemia of mixed phenotype with t (9; 22) (q34; q11.2); BCR-ABL 1 Acute leukemia of phenotype mixed with t (v; 11q23); MLL rearrangement Acute leukemia, mixed phenotype, B/myeloid, and NOS Acute mixed phenotype leukemia, T/myeloid, and NOS Acute mixed phenotype leukemia, and NOS—rare types Other leukemias of ambiguous lineage

Source: Adapted from Vardiman (2008)

dose according to the actual weight of the pregnant woman and adjusting it according to her weight gain during pregnancy is a coherent conduct [5].

The successful treatment for acute myeloid leukemia is in its systemic elimination and through the bone marrow—and thus, consequently, restoration of normal hematopoiesis. In this type of leukemia, the infiltration of the disease by the central nervous system (CNS) affects a small rate of affected patients—around 5%—so its treatment is not carried out prophylactically and routinely [11].

Table 3.3 Chemotherapy protocols for AML

Protocol	Treatment	Emetogenic potential	Reference
Ara-C + Daunorubicin (3 + 7)	Cytarabine: 100 mg/m²/day continuous IV from D1 to D7 Daunorubicin: 90 mg/m² IV from D1 to D3	Moderate	Fernandez H, et al. Anthracycline Dose Intensification in Acute Myeloid Leukemia. N Engl J Med 2009; 361:1249–1259
Ara-C + Daunorubicin	Cytarabine: 100 mg/m²/12 h IV from D1 to D10 Daunorubicin: 60 mg/m²/day IV infusion of D1, D3, and D5	–	Ali S, et al. Guidelines for the diagnosis and management of acute myeloid leukaemia in pregnancy. British Journal of Haematology 2015; 170: 487–495
Ara-C + idarubicin (3 + 7)	Cytarabine: 100 mg/m²/day continuous IV from D1 to D7 Idarubicin: 12 mg/m² IV from D1 to D3	Moderate	Preisler H, et al. Comparison of three remission induction regimens and two postinduction strategies for the treatment of acute nonlymphocytic leukemia: a Cancer Leukemia Group B study. Blood 1987; 69:1441–1449.
Ara-C + Idarubicin + Cladribine (7 + 3 + 5)	Idarubicin: 12 mg/m² IV from D1 to D3. Cytarabine: 200 mg/m² IV from D1 to D7 Cladribine: 5 mg/m² IV from D1 to D5	Moderate	Holowiecki J, et al. Cladribine in Combination with Standard Daunorubicine and Cytarabine (DAC) as a Remission Induction Treatment Improves the Overall Survival in Untreated Adults with AML Aged < 60 y Contrary to Combination Including Fludarabine (DAF): A Multicenter, Randomized, Phase III PALG AML 1/2004 DAC/DAF/DA Study in 673 Patients-A Final Update. Blood 2009;114:Abstract 2055.

(continued)

Table 3.3 (continued)

Protocol	Treatment	Emetogenic potential	Reference
High-dose cytarabine	Cytarabine: 3000 mg/m² IV in 3 hours, every 12 hours in D1, D3, and D5 Cytarabine: 1500 mg/m² IV in 3 hours, every 12 hours in D1, D3, and D5	Moderate	Mayer RJ, et al. Intensive postremission chemotherapy in adults with acute myeloid leukemia. Cancer and leukemia Group B. N Engl J Med 1994;331:896–903. Burnett AK, et al. Attempts to Optimise Induction and Consolidation Chemotherapy in Patients with Acute Myeloid Leukaemia: Results of the MRC AML15 Trial. Blood 2009;114: Abstract 484.
MIDAM (Ara-C and Mitoxantrone)	Cytarabine: 1000 mg/m² IV in 2 hours, every 12 hours from D1 to D5 Mitoxantrone: 12 mg/m² IV from D1 to D3	Moderate	Chevallier P, et al. Long Term Disease Free Survival after Gemtuzumab, Intermediate-Dose Cytarabine and Mitoxantrone in patients with CD33+ Primary Resistant or Relapsed Acute Myeloid Leukemia. J Clin Oncol 2008;26:5192–5197.
FLAG	Fludarabine: 30 mg/m² IV in 30 minutes from D1 to D5. Cytarabine: 2000 mg/m² IV in 4 hours from D1 to D5. Filgrastim: 5 mcg/kg SC from D1 to D5	Moderate	Borthakur G., et al. Treatment of Core-Binding Factor in Acute Myelogenous Leukemia with Fludarabine, Cytarabine and Granulocyte Colony-stimulating factor results in improved event-free survival. Cancer 2008;113:3181–5.

Table 3.3 (continued)

Protocol	Treatment	Emetogenic potential	Reference
CLAG-M	Cladribine: 5 mg/m² IV in 2 hours from D1 to D5 Cytarabine: 2000 mg/m² IV in 4 hours from D1 to D5, starting at 2 hours after the end of cladribine Mitoxantrone: 120 mg/m² IV from D1 to D3 Filgrastim: 600 mcg/day IV from D0 to D5	Moderate	Wierzbowska A, et al. Cladribine combined with high doses of arabinoside cytosine, mitoxantrone, and G-CSF (CLAG-M) is a highly effective salvage regimen in patients with refractory and relapsed acute myeloid leukemia of the poor risk: a final report of the Polish Adult Leukemia Group. Eur J Haematol 2007;80:115–126.
MEC	Etoposide: 80 mg/m² IV in 1 hour. Cytarabine: 1000 mg/m² IV in 6 hours after etoposide Mitoxantrone: 6 mg/m² IV in bolus after cytarabine from D1 to D6	Moderate	Amadori S, et al. Mitoxantrone, Etoposide, and Intermediate-Dose Cytarabine: An Effective and Tolerable Regimen for the Treatment of Refractory Acute Myeloid Leukemia. J Clin Oncol 1991;9:1210–1214.
Cyclophosphamide + Etoposide	Etoposide: 2400 mg/m² IV in continuous infusion for 34 hours in D1 and D2. Cyclophosphamide: 2000 mg/m² IV in 3 hours from D3 to D5	Moderate	Johny A, et al. Early Stem Cell Transplantation for Refractory Acute Leukemia after Salvage Therapy with Etoposide and Cyclophosphamide. Biol Blood Marrow Transplant 2006;12:480–489.
Decitabine	Decitabine: 20 mg/m² IV in 1 hour from D1 to D10. Repeat the cycle every 28 days	Minimum	Blum W, et al. Clinical response and mir-29b predictive significance in older AML patients treated with a 10-day schedule of decitabine. Proc National Acad Sci 2010;107:7473–7478.

3.2.2 Acute Promyelocytic Leukemia

Acute promyelocytic leukemia is like a subtype of acute myeloid leukemia and although its incidence is not precisely known, including cases in pregnant women, APL is a relatively rare hematological neoplasm. The general numbers of newly diagnosed cases in the United States reach approximately 600–800 per year [12]. This leukemia preferably affects the age group from 20 years to 59 years, that is, mainly in the age group of young adults, when compared to the other subtypes of AML—this period corresponds to a large part of the female reproductive period [13]. Suspected APL should be considered a medical emergency, which requires several simultaneous actions, such as the introduction of therapy with all-trans-retinoic acid (ATRA; tretinoin), genetic diagnosis, and measures to neutralize coagulopathy [12].

ATRA is a natural metabolite, derived from retinol, belonging to the family of retinoids, which is able to act on the bone marrow, through cell differentiation therapy, promoting the process of cell pro-apoptosis, and inhibiting the growth of leukemic cells. This treatment is able to increase patient survival by up to 80% and shows remission of the disease by up to 90%. However, about 5–20% of patients treated with ATRA develop a type of severe reaction to the drug called APL differentiation syndrome, which is considered a very serious reaction and has important mortality rates. For this, studies have been developed, in order to avoid it through delivery systems, as, for example, in nanocapsules, which, together with the drug, significantly improve the issue of toxicity so worrying in the context of the pregnant woman's health [13].

According to a panel of experts on behalf of European LeukemiaNet (2009), which addresses a topic on clinical management in pregnant women diagnosed with acute promyelocytic leukemia, treatment is approached according to the necessary care involved in each trimester of pregnancy. Thus, ATRA and arsenic trioxide (ATO) therapy should be avoided in the first trimester of pregnancy due to their teratogenic potential. Arsenic trioxide (ATO), as it is embryotoxic, is not recommended at any stage of pregnancy, and ATRA therapy has the potential for the development of fetal malformations and spontaneous abortion in the first trimester. The panel's therapeutic decision is to follow the chemotherapy use of anthracycline if the pregnant woman continues with the pregnancy. Of the suggested anthracyclines, daunorubicin is preferable because it is an agent with more efficacy proven by the use of pregnant women with APL and by scientific records. On the contrary, there are doubts about the use of idarubicin—a more lipolytic agent—and that, therefore, would have a greater chance of overcoming the placental barrier. In the following trimesters of gestation, APL may be treated with ATRA therapy; however, with a caveat about fetal monitoring, particularly of cardiac function, although the treatment is relatively safe, and with anthracycline-based chemotherapy [12].

3.2.3 Acute Lymphoid Leukemia (ALL)

Acute lymphoid leukemia (ALL) is the most common type of cancer in children, constituting about one-third of all malignant neoplasms in children [14]. The treatment of ALL is long, ranging from 2 years to 3 years. Although the therapeutic regimens can change from center to center, the current protocols are formed by five phases: induction of remission, intensification-consolidation, reinduction, prevention of leukemia in the central nervous system (CNS), and continuation or maintenance of remission [15]. Following current treatment protocols, more than 80% of disease remission is achieved. However, only about 40% of adults will be alive 2 years after the start of treatment, unlike children, who tend to have a survival rate of more than 80% [11].

The development of therapeutic combinations using various cytotoxic drugs, with or without stem-cell transplantation, has increased the percentage of cure for ALL patients by more than 80% [16]. This evidence of improved results has produced an increase in the population of ALL survivors. It is currently estimated that one in 1000 young adults, under the age of 20, is a cancer survivor. Therefore, late complications represent another area of possible investment, in addition to the importance of planning the initial treatment to avoid such complications [17].

Therefore, the chemotherapy protocols used for ALL in pregnant women and children can be those described in Table 3.4.

In general, success in the treatment of acute lymphoid leukemia is in the elimination of bone marrow disease and its systemic infiltration. However, it is known that leukemic cells may not be completely eliminated, causing relapses that compromise the survival of affected patients [11].

3.3 Chronic Leukemia

Chronic leukemias are presentations with a rarer incidence than acute leukemias during pregnancy. In part, one can consider the fact that its incidence accompanies the progressive increase in age—in this way, its diagnosis happens around the age of 45–50, which does not normally correspond to the female reproductive age [3].

Chronic lymphoid leukemia-B presents symptoms between 55 years and 65 years, is extremely rare under the age of 30 and is approximately twice as common in men [11].

Table 3.4 Chemotherapy protocols for ALL

Hyper-CVAD

Induction	Treatment	Emetogenic potential for induction	Anaphylactic potential
Patient room with laminar flow if aged >60 years	Rituximab: 375 mg/m² IV on D1 and D11 (odd cycle) or on D1 and D8 (even cycle) if leukemic blasts with ≥20% expression for a total of eight doses (four first cycles) and during intensifications in months 6 and 18 of the treatment.	Moderate	Moderate with rituximab

Maintenance (for 30 months)

Protocol	Treatment	Emetogenic potential	Anaphylactic potential
POMP (Months 1–5, 8–17 and 20–30)	Prednisone: 200 mg orally from D1 to D5 monthly. Vincristine: 2 mg IV on D1 monthly. Methotrexate: 20 mg/m² IV weekly. Mercaptopurine: 150 mg/day orally. Administer at night. Adjust methotrexate and mercaptopurine dose as needed to maintain leukocytes between 2000/mm³ and 3000/mm³ and for liver toxicity.	Minimum for intravenous drugs.	
Hyper-CVAD ± rituximab (Months 6 e 18)	Cyclophosphamide: 300 mg/m² IV in 3 hours and every 12 hours for six doses from D1 to D3 (Hospital MD Anderson protocol suggests infusion in 3 hours). Mesna: 600 mg/m² IV in 24 hours from D1 to D3, ending 6 hours after the last dose of cyclophosphamide. Vincristine: 2 mg IV on D4 and D11. Doxorubicin: 50 mg/m² IV in 24 hours on D4. Dexamethasone: 40 mg orally or IV from D1 to D4 and from D11 to D14. Rituximab: 375 mg/m² IV D1 and D11 if leukemic blasts with CD20 expression ≥20%.	Moderate	Moderate with rituximab
Methotrexate and Asparaginase (Months 7 and 19)	Methotrexate: 100 mg/m² IV on D1, D8, D15, and D22. Asparaginase: 20,000 IU/m² IV weekly on D2, D9, D16, and D23	Low	

GRAAL-2003		
Corticosteroid pre-phase		
Prednisone: 60 mg/m² orally from D-7 to D-1.		
Methotrexate: 15 mg IT from D-7 to D-4.		
Protocol	*Treatment*	*Emetogenic potential for induction*	*Recommendations*
Induction	Prednisone: 60 mg/m² orally from D1 to D14. Daunorubicin: 50 mg/m²/day from D1 to D3. Daunorubicin: 30 mg/m²/day on D15 and D16. Vincristine: 2 mg IV on D1, D8, D15 and D22. Asparaginase: 6000 IU/m²/day on D8, D10, D12, D20, D22, D24, D26, and D28. Cyclophosphamide: 750 mg/m²/day on D1. Cyclophosphamide: 750 mg/m²/day at D15 (B-ALL and good responders). Cyclophosphamide: 500 mg/m² IV 12/12 h on D15 and D16 (T-ALL or bad responders). Filgrastim: 300 mcg SC or IV from D17 until neutrophil recovery.	Moderate	Check recommendations for prevention of nausea and vomiting of oral agents.
Rescue for those who did not go into full remission after induction	Idarubicin: 12 mg/m² from D1 to D3. Cytarabine: 2000 mg/m² IV 12/12 h from D1 to D4. Filgrastim: 300 mcg SC or IV from D9 until neutrophil recovery. Prophylaxis of cytarabine conjunctivitis. 0.1% dexamethasone eye drops: one drop in each eye, 4–6 times a day.	Moderate	

(continued)

Table 3.4 (continued)

| Consolidation | Consolidation consists of nine blocks of therapy administered every 2 weeks, with some modifications to the schedule due to hematological recovery. Late intensification is administered between blocks 6 and 7. Allogeneic transplantation is performed after blocks 3 or 6, depending on the availability of the donor.

Blocks 1, 4, and 7:
Cytarabine: 2000 mg/m² IV 12/12 h in D1 and D2.
Dexamethasone: 10 mg VO 12/12 h no D1 e D2.
Asparaginase: 10,000 IU/m² in D3.
Filgrastim: 300 mcg from D7 to D13.
Prophylaxis of cytarabine conjunctivitis.
0.1% dexamethasone eye drops: one drop in each eye, 4–6 times a day.
Blocks 2, 5, and 8:
Methotrexate—3000 mg/m² IV in a 24-h continuous infusion pump at D15.
Calcium folinate: 15 mg IV 6/6 h for eight doses, starting 12 hours after completion.
methotrexate; dose changes based on methotrexate levels.
Vincristine: 2 mg IV on D15.
Asparaginase: 10,000 IU/m² in D16.
Mercaptopurine: 60 mg/m²/day from D15 to D21.
Filgrastim: 300 mcg from D22 to D27.
Blocks 3, 6, and 9:
Cyclophosphamide—500 mg/m² IV on D29 and D30.
Etoposide: 75 mg/m² IV on D29 and D30.
Methotrexate: 25 mg/m² IV on D29.
Filgrastim: 300 mcg from D31 until neutrophil recovery. | Moderate (for all blocks) |

Late intensification (administer between blocks 6 and 7)	For patients in complete remission after the first induction cycle. Prednisone: 60 mg/m²/day VO from D1 to D14. Vincristine: 2 mg IV on D1, D8, and D15. Daunorubicin: 30 mg/m² from D1 to D3. Asparaginase: 6000 IU/m²/day in D8, D10, D12, D18, D20, and D22. Cyclophosphamide: 500 mg/m² IV 12/12 h on D15. Filgrastim: 300 mcg when neutrophils < 500/mm³, until neutrophil recovery. For patients in complete remission after rescue. Idarubicin: 9 mg/m² IV from D1 to D3. Cytarabine: 2000 mg/m² IV 12/12 h from D1 to D4. Filgrastim: 300 mcg SC or IV from D9 until neutrophil recovery. Prophylaxis of cytarabine conjunctivitis. 0.1% dexamethasone eye drops: one drop in each eye, 4—6 times a day.	Moderate	
Maintenance (for 24 months after consolidation ends)	Prednisone: 40 mg/m²/day orally from D1 to D7. Vincristine: 2 mg IV on D1. Repeat the cycle every 28 days, for a total of 12 cycles. Methotrexate: 25 mg/m² orally weekly for 24 months. Mercaptopurine: 60 mg/m²/day orally for 24 months.	Minimum for intravenous.		Check recommendations for prevention of nausea and vomiting of oral agents.
Hyper-CVAD			
Induction	*Treatment*	*Emetogenic potential for induction*	*Anaphylactic potential*
Patient room with laminar flow if aged >60 years	Rituximab: 375 mg/m² IV on D1 and D11 (odd cycle) or on D1 and D8 (even cycle) if leukemic blasts with ≥20% expression for a total of 8 doses (4 first cycles) and during intensifications in months 6 and 18 of the treatment.	Moderate	Moderate with rituximab

(continued)

Table 3.4 (continued)

Maintenance (for 30 months)

Protocol	Treatment	Emetogenic potential	Anaphylactic potential
POMP (Months 1–5, 8–17 and 20–30)	Prednisone: 200 mg orally from D1 to D5 monthly. Vincristine: 2 mg IV on D1 monthly. Methotrexate: 20 mg/m^2 IV weekly. Mercaptopurine: 150 mg/day orally. Administer at night. Adjust methotrexate and mercaptopurine dose as needed to maintain leukocytes between 2000–3000/mm^3 and for liver toxicity.	Minimum for intravenous drugs.	
Hyper-CVAD ± rituximab (Meses 6 e 18)	Cyclophosphamide: 300 mg/m^2 IV in 3 hours every 12 hours for six doses from D1 to D3 (Hospital MD Anderson protocol suggests infusion in 3 hours). medicine: 600 mg/m^2 IV in 24 hours from D1 to D3, ending 6 hours after the last dose of cyclophosphamide. Vincristine: 2 mg IV on D4 and D11. Doxorubicin: 50 mg/m^2 IV in 24 hours on D4. Dexamethasone: 40 mg orally or IV from D1 to D4 and from D11 to D14. Rituximab: 375 mg/m^2 IV D1 and D11 if leukemic blasts with CD20 expression ≥20%.	Moderate	Médio com rituximab
Methotrexate and Asparaginase (Months 7 and 19)	Methotrexate: 100 mg/m^2 IV on D1, D8, D15 and D22. Asparaginase: 20,000 IU/m^2 IV weekly on D2, D9, D16 and D23	Low	

GRAAL-2003			
Corticosteroid pre-phase			
Prednisone: 60 mg/m² orally from D7 to D1. Methotrexate: 15 mg IT from D7 to D4.			
Protocol	*Treatment*	*Emetogenic potential for induction*	*recommendations*
Induction	Prednisone: 60 mg/m² orally from D1 to D14. Daunorubicin: 50 mg/m²/day from D1 to D3. Daunorubicin: 30 mg/m²/day on D15 and D16. Vincristine: 2 mg IV on D1, D8, D15, and D22. Asparaginase: 6000 IU/m²/day on D8, D10, D12, D20, D22, D24, D26 and D28. Cyclophosphamide: 750 mg/m²/day on D1. Cyclophosphamide: 750 mg/m²/day at D15 (B-ALL and good responders). Cyclophosphamide: 500 mg/m² IV 12/12 h on D15 and D16 (T-ALL or bad responders). Filgrastim: 300 mcg SC or IV from D17 until neutrophil recovery	Moderate	Check recommendations for prevention of nausea and vomiting of oral agents.
Rescue for those who did not go into full remission after induction	Idarubicin: 12 mg/m² from D1 to D3. Cytarabine: 2000 mg/m² IV 12/12 h from D1 to D4. Filgrastim: 300 mcg SC or IV from D9 until neutrophil recovery. Prophylaxis of cytarabine conjunctivitis. 0.1% dexamethasone eye drops: one drop in each eye, 4–6 times a day.	Moderate	

(continued)

Table 3.4 (continued)

Consolidation	Consolidation consists of 9 blocks of therapy administered every 2 weeks, with some modifications to the schedule due to hematological recovery. Late intensification is administered between blocks 6 and 7. Allogeneic transplantation is performed after blocks 3 or 6, depending on the availability of the donor.	Moderate (for all blocks)

Blocks 1, 4 and 7:
Cytarabine: 2000 mg/m^2 IV 12/12 h in D1 and D2.
Dexamethasone: 10 mg VO 12/12 h no D1 e D2.
Asparaginase: 10,000 IU/m^2 in D3.
Filgrastim: 300 mcg from D7 to D13.
Prophylaxis of cytarabine conjunctivitis.
0.1% dexamethasone eye drops: one drop in each eye, 4 to 6 times a day.

Blocks 2, 5 and 8:
Methotrexate: 3000 mg/m^2 IV in a 24-hour continuous infusion pump at D15.
Calcium folinate: 15 mg IV 6/6 h for 8 doses, starting 12 hours after completion. methotrexate; dose changes based on methotrexate levels.
Vincristine: 2 mg IV on D15.
Asparaginase: 10,000 IU/m^2 in D16.
Mercaptopurine: 60 mg/m^2/day from D15 to D21.
Filgrastim: 300 mcg from D22 to D27

Blocks 3, 6 and 9:
Cyclophosphamide: 500 mg/m^2 IV on D29 and D30.
Etoposide: 75 mg/m^2 IV on D29 and D30.
Methotrexate: 25 mg/m^2 IV on D29.
Filgrastim: 300 mcg from D31 until neutrophil recovery.

| Late intensification (administer between blocks 6 and 7) | For patients in complete remission after the first induction cycle. Prednisone: 60 mg/m²/day VO from D1 to D14. Vincristine: 2 mg IV on D1, D8 and D15. Daunorubicin: 30 mg/m² from D1 to D3. Asparaginase: 6000 IU/m²/day in D8, D10, D12, D18, D20 and D22. Cyclophosphamide: 500 mg/m² IV 12/12 h on D15. Filgrastim: 300 mcg when neutrophils <500/mm³, until neutrophil recovery. For patients in complete remission after rescue. Idarubicin: 9 mg/m² IV from D1 to D3. Cytarabine: 2000 mg/m² IV 12/12 h from D1 to D4. Filgrastim: 300 mcg SC or IV from D9 until neutrophil recovery. Prophylaxis of cytarabine conjunctivitis. 0.1% dexamethasone eye drops: one drop in each eye, 4–6 times a day. | Moderate | |
| Maintenance (for 24 months after consolidation ends) | Prednisone: 40 mg/m²/day orally from D1 to D7. Vincristine: 2 mg IV on D1. Repeat the cycle every 28 days, for a total of 12 cycles. Methotrexate: 25 mg/m² orally weekly for 24 months. Mercaptopurine: 60 mg/m²/day orally for 24 months. | Minimum for intravenous. | Check recommendations for prevention of nausea and vomiting of oral agents. |

Source: Thomas et al. [24]

3.3.1 Chronic Myeloid Leukemia

Chronic myeloid leukemia (CML) is a myeloproliferative disease characterized by excessive accumulation of normal-looking myeloid cells. It occurs with an annual incidence of 1.0–1.5 per 100,000 inhabitants, affecting mainly adults, between 50 years and 55 years of age. In Brazil, in 2012, 81,100 CML chemotherapy procedures were recorded in the SUS Outpatient Information System (SIA-SUS), indicating an annual incidence of 10,125 cases of this disease [7]. The clinical picture can be presented with marked splenomegaly and increased leukometries, but with the functions of neutrophils preserved [3].

CML is characterized by the presence of the Philadelphia chromosome (Ph+) and the oncogene that encodes it, present in most myeloid cells and in some lymphocytes. CML is comprised of three phases [18]: chronic initial and progressive phase (average duration of 4–5 years), transformation phase (accelerated) of variable duration depending on each individual's organism, and terminal phase called blast phase (acute) [19].

Clinical management in the treatment of chronic myeloid leukemia consists of a complex process, since antineoplastic therapy can be harmful to the mother and the fetus due to the potential harmful effect. However, pregnancy does not seem to alter the course of CML, and, depending on the case, treatment does not need to be started immediately. However, it should be noted that CML may favor the risk of placental insufficiency and, therefore, low birth weight, increased rates of prematurity, perinatal morbidity, and mortality [3].

Conventional chemotherapy for CML consists of hydroxyurea; busulfan (inhibitors of DNA synthesis)—inexpensive compounds that bring few adverse events, but have the potential to cause miscarriage; fetal growth restriction; and congenital malformations; interferon-alfa-2b with more frequent adverse effects; and lately, a tyrosine kinase inhibitor—imatinib mesylate—has been used, which despite the teratogenic effect, case reports have shown use without fetal involvement [3].

Therefore, the chemotherapy protocols used for CML in pregnant women and adult individuals can be those described in Table 3.5.

The Ministry of Health of Brazil, through the Health Care Secretariat (2008), presents data regarding the results of patients undergoing chemotherapy in different stages of CML. The chronic phase of CML may have its peripheral manifestations contained in the application of oral chemotherapy with, for example, busulfan or hydroxyurea—however, such control does not alter the course of CML. Patients who received alpha interferon as chemotherapy in the chronic phase had an overall survival of 67% in 5 years and 40% in 10 years. Patients who received imatinib mesylate, as their first treatment, achieved 76% complete cytogenetic response and, of these, 90% had an overall survival of around 54 months. Among those who did not receive treatment with imatinib mesylate as a first line, 41–64% had a complete cytogenetic response, of which 86–88% had an overall half-life of 4 years. However, there are still restrictions in these comparisons between the use of alpha interferon and the use of imatinib because the use is based on historical data [19].

Table 3.5 Chemotherapy protocols for CML

Protocol	Treatment	Emetogenic potential	Reference
Imatinib	Imatinib: 400 mg/day orally.	Check recommendations for prevention of nausea and vomiting of oral agents.	*Kantarjian H, et al. Hematologic and Cytogenetic Responses to Imatinib Mesylate in Chronic Myelogenous Leukemia. NEJM.2002;346:645–52.361:1249–1259*
Dasatinib	Dasatinib: 70 mg orally two times a day. Dasatinib: 100 mg orally/day.	Check recommendations for prevention of nausea and vomiting of oral agents.	*Shah NP; et al. Intermittent target inhibition with dasatinib 100 mg once daily preserves efficacy and improves tolerability in imatinib-resistant and -intolerant chronic-phase chronic myeloid leukemia. J Clin Oncol. 2008;26 (19):3204–12.*
Nilotinib	Nilotinib: 400 mg orally two times a day.	Check recommendations for prevention of nausea and vomiting of oral agents.	*Available from the US FDA website at:* www.fda.gov/cder/foi/label/2007/022068lbl.pdf.
Hydroxyurea	Hydroxyurea: 40 mg/kg/day orally.	Check recommendations for prevention of nausea and vomiting of oral agents.	*Hehlmann R, et al. Randomized comparison of interferon-alpha with busulfan and hydroxyurea in chronic myelogenous leukemia. The German CML Study Group. Blood 1994;84:4064–4077.*
Alpha interferon 2nd	Alfa interferon 2nd 5,000,000 IU/m²/day SC. Start with 2000,000 IU/m²/day three times a week and increase as tolerated.	Minimum	*Kantarjian HM, O'Brien S, Cortes JE, et al. Complete cytogenetic and molecular responses to interferon alpha based therapy for chronic myelogenous leukemia are associated with excellent long-term prognosis. Cancer. 2003;97 (4):1033.*

In the transformation phase of CML, the Ministry of Health noted that patients who received imatinib mesylate during this ongoing phase of CML had approximately 19% complete cytogenetic response, and 40% remained without leukemic progression for a duration of 3 years. The blast phase is more aggressive and tends to be more resistant to treatment. As a result of this condition, the patient's survival is around 3–5 months, while those who received treatment with imatinib mesylate obtained the disease progression for less than 10 months, and only 7% were alive after 3 years [19].

Lopes, Lyeyasu, and Castro (2008) state that the introduction of tyrosine kinase inhibitors has revolutionized the treatment of chronic myeloid leukemia considerably, due to its effectiveness in the hematological and cytogenetic control of the disease. In their phase III clinical study, two groups of patients were separated by chemotherapy received. One group received imatinib mesylate as a chemotherapy treatment, against the other that received interferon plus Ara-C. The group that corresponded to chemotherapy with imatinib mesylate demonstrated rapid attainment of the hematological response, with the following results: hemoglobin concentration greater than 10 g/dl and number of leukocytes and platelets less than $10 \times 10^3/$ mm^3 and $500 \times 10^3/mm^3$, respectively. In addition, the effectiveness of imatinib mesylate in promoting cytogenetic and molecular responses in a short period of time has been demonstrated. This results in disease control in more than 87% of treated patients [11].

However, the Ministry of Health still notes that according to national and international experiences with the use of imatinib mesylate, it has no curative potential for chronic myeloid leukemia. In about 5 years, 40% of patients who were in the chronic phase and 60% of those who were in the transformation phase gained resistance to treatment with imatinib mesylate. In those who received it in the blast phase, 100% showed resistance in the first year of treatment; the best response to CML was with those in the chronic phase who used dasatinib (another tyrosine kinase inhibitor) in a study conducted in 139 health centers with follow-up of more than 650 patients. In this case, dasatinib proved to be 365 times more potent in vitro than imatinib: it provided a complete hematological response in 90% of patients with a cytogenetic response greater than 59%, a complete cytogenetic response of 43%, and progression-free survival of 83% in 12 months. This study also included 157 patients of CML in the blast phase, with an overall survival (24 months of follow-up) of 26% in the lymphoid-type LMC and 36% in the myeloid type [19].

Regarding the use of nilotinib (NIL) in pregnant women, specifically with chronic myeloid leukemia, 11 women were treated with tyrosine kinase inhibitors for an average of 56 (20–113) months before pregnancy, of which treatment with NIL was approximately 34 (3–48) months on average. Of the 12 pregnancies that occurred, 10 pregnancies were unique, and 1 pregnancy was double, of which 9 patients received NIL at 600 mg/day in early pregnancy and 1 case with exposure to NIL at 800 mg/day (mean time of treatments was 4–6 weeks). Of the eight pregnancies that resulted in delivery, five resulted in the birth of well-developed babies, two had spontaneous abortion, and there was a case of a baby with syndactyly deformity, whose mother was exposed to NIL A 600 mg/day for 7 weeks at the very beginning of the trimester of pregnancy [20].

3.4 Final Considerations About Chemotherapy Applied in Pregnancy Complicated by Leukemia

Clinical management in choosing the chemotherapy treatment for leukemia, in general, generates doubts and distress on the part of the health professionals responsible for making the decision regarding the indication of chemotherapy and the monitoring of a patient. Thus, when the theme is approached within the demanding clinical conditions of a pregnant woman, the complexity of this clinical decision is greatly increased.

Considering the maternal and fetal risks associated with the most prevalent types of leukemias in pregnant women, the approach of Nomura et al. (2011) that acute leukemias affect pregnant women can favor an outcome for maternal morbidity and adverse perinatal results. Therefore, in these conditions, clinical management should be monitoring of hematological abnormalities, in order to prepare the pregnant woman for delivery. In chronic myeloid leukemia, maternal and fetal prognoses seem to be more favorable, with easier intervention in possible complications [3].

Table 3.6 gathers data from the study that carried out a survey on the data regarding the complications observed in 16 pregnant women affected by acute leukemias (AML and ALL) and chronic myeloid leukemia (CML), relating them to their respective antineoplastic treatments and supportive or additional therapies.

Thus, although other factors are related to the emergence of complications during pregnancy with leukemia and not only with isolated pharmacological therapies—chemotherapy or additional as emphasized here, such as the gestational period in which these women were when they started receiving chemotherapy treatment and additional treatment not mentioned here—it is important that the professional responsible for monitoring this pregnant woman is attentive to the potential reactions that chemotherapeutic drugs can trigger. The following are briefly the possible adverse reactions of the main chemotherapy drugs used by pregnant women in this process.

3.4.1 Cytarabine

As cytarabine is a bone marrow suppressor; the expected reactions may be anemia, leukopenia, thrombocytopenia, megaloblastosis, and reduced reticulocytes as a result of administration. The severity of these reactions depends on the dose and the therapeutic regimen employed. Cellular changes in morphology can also be expected in smears of bone marrow and peripheral blood. Regarding infectious

Table 3.6 Therapeutic characteristics used in pregnant women complicated by leukemia

Case	Disease	Antineoplastic therapy in pregnancy	Additional therapy	Maternal complications
1[a]	ALL	–	–	Thrombocytopenia
2[a]	ALL	–	–	Thrombocytopenia
3	ALL	Cytarabine, daunorubicin, and vincristine	Prednisone, allopurinol, and granulokine	Anemia and thrombocytopenia
4[b]	ALL	Cyclophosphamide and vincristine	Prednisone, vancomycin, tazobactam, and granulokine	Anemia, thrombocytopenia, and febrile neutropenia
5[c]	ALL	–	Ceftriaxone, clindamycin, imipenem, vancomycin, and granulokine	Tooth abscess, anemia, and thrombocytopenia, febrile neutropenia
6	AML	Citarabin and daunorubicina	Dexamethasone, vancomycin, piperacillin, and tazobactam	Anemia, thrombocytopenia, and febrile neutropenia
7	AML	Cytarabine, daunorubicin, and all-transretinoic acid	Dexamethasone, vancomycin, and metronidazole	Anemia, thrombocytopenia, febrile neutropenia, infection, and scar hematoma
8	CML	Imatinib up to 10 weeks	–	Urinary infection
9	CML	Imatinib up to 12 weeks	Granulokine and nitrofurantoin	Urinary infection
10	CML	Imatinib up to 25 weeks	–	No
11	CML	Interferon	–	Scar infection
12	CML	Interferon	–	No
13	CML	Interferon	Plaquetopheresis	No
14	CML	Hydroxyurea (18 weeks to 20 weeks), interferon	–	No
15	CML	Hydroxyurea	–	No
16	CML	Imatinib (up to 8 weeks), interferon and leukopheresis, hydroxyurea	–	No

Source: Namura et al. [25]
ALL acute lymphoid leukemia, *AML* acute myeloid leukemia, *CML* chronic myeloid leukemia
[a]Therapeutic abortion
[b]Maternal death 6 months after delivery
[c]Late diagnosis and therapy initiated after delivery

complications, the patient is prone to viral, bacterial, fungal, or parasitic infections anywhere on the body, through the use of Aracytin® (cytarabine) alone or combined with other immunosuppressive agents after immunosuppressive doses that affect cellular immunity or humerus.

These infections can not only be mild but also serious and even fatal. Castleberry (1981) described a cytarabine syndrome: fever, myalgia, bone pain, occasionally chest pain, maculopapular rash, conjunctivitis, and malaise. It usually occurs 6–12 hours after drug administration. Corticosteroids have been shown to be beneficial in the treatment or prevention of this syndrome. If symptoms are considered treatable, the use of corticosteroids should be considered, as well as continued therapy with Aracytin®.

The most frequent adverse reactions are nausea, anorexia, vomiting, diarrhea, liver dysfunction, fever, rashes, thrombophlebitis, oral and anal inflammation or ulceration, and bleeding. Nausea and vomiting are more frequent after administration by rapid intravenous injection.

3.4.2 Daunorubicin

Among the complications and reactions noted for daunorubicin are sepsis/septicemia, infection, bone marrow failure, leukopenia, granulocytopenia, neutropenia, thrombocytopenia, and anemia.

3.4.3 Cyclophosphamide

Cyclophosphamide includes cardiac reactions such as cardiac arrest, ventricular fibrillation, ventricular tachycardia, cardiogenic shock, pericardial effusion (progressing to cardiac tamponade), myocardial hemorrhage, myocardial infarction, heart failure (including fatal outcomes), cardiomyopathy, myocarditis, cardiac disease, pericarditis, atrial fibrillation, supraventricular arrhythmia, ventricular arrhythmia, bradycardia, tachycardia, palpitations, and QT prolongation; ear and labyrinth reactions: deafness, hearing loss, and tinnitus; congenital, familiar, and genetic reactions: intrauterine death, fetal malformation, fetal growth retardation, and fetal toxicity (including myelosuppression, gastroenteritis).

3.4.4 Vincristine

When using vincristine, there is a risk of acute uric nephropathy, leukopenia, or infection with complications. In this case, a complete blood count should be taken before the next dose is administered. There may be neurological changes and use of neurotoxic drugs (e.g., disulfiram) to avoid possible adverse reactions, liver failure (liver problems), jaundice (yellowish skin color), liver radiation, neuromuscular disease, and lung problems.

3.4.5   All-Trans-Retinoic Acid

All-trans-retinoic acid can trigger adverse skin reactions such as dryness, erythema, rash, itching, sweating, and hair loss. Genital ulceration and Sweet's syndrome have been reported infrequently. Erythema nodosum has been reported rarely. In mucous membranes, reactions such as cheilitis; dry mouth; and nose, conjunctiva, and other mucous membranes with or without inflammatory symptoms were noted. In the central nervous system, headache, intracranial hypertension/cerebral pseudotumor (mainly in children), fever, tremors, dizziness, confusion, anxiety, depression, paraesthesia, insomnia, and malaise have been reported. In the neurosensory system, vision and hearing disorders can occur. In the musculoskeletal system, bone and chest pain may occur, in addition to reported myositis in rare cases. In the gastrointestinal tract, nausea, vomiting, abdominal pain, constipation, diarrhea, decreased appetite, and pancreatitis are reported. Regarding metabolic, hepatic, and renal dysfunctions, reactions such as triglyceride levels, cholesterol, transaminases (ALT, AST), and serum creatinine are present. Occasional cases of hypercalcemia have been reported. In the respiratory system, dyspnea, respiratory failure, pleural effusion, and asthma-like syndrome are reported. In the cardiovascular system, arrhythmias, flushing, and edema are reported. Some cases of thrombosis involving multiple sites have been reported infrequently. Finally, hematological reactions such as thrombocytes have been reported rarely; marked basophilia with or without symptomatic hyperhistaminemia has been reported rarely, especially in patients with a rare variation of APL associated with basophilic differentiation.

3.4.6   Imatinib

The most frequent adverse reactions to the drug included gastrointestinal bleeding, conjunctivitis, and elevated transaminases or bilirubin. Other adverse reactions to the drug were reported less or equal, although the adverse reactions described in the package insert occurred in patients who escalated the dose to 800 mg—which is not the case for the indication for pregnant women as exemplified in the text.

3.4.7   Hydroxyurea

The known adverse reactions are leukopenia, anemia, and thrombocytopenia; stomatitis, anorexia, nausea, vomiting, diarrhea, and constipation; maculopapular rash, facial erythema, peripheral erythema, skin ulceration, and skin changes such as dermatomyositis. Hyperpigmentation of the nails, atrophy of the skin and nails, peeling, violet papules and alopecia were observed in some patients after several years of daily maintenance therapy with hydroxyurea. Azoospermia, oligospermia, bone marrow failure, decrease in CD4 lymphocytes, pancreatitis, mucositis, stomach discomfort, dyspepsia, skin vasculitis, papular rash, skin exfoliation, skin atrophy, skin ulcer, skin hyperpigmentation; dysuria, increased blood creatinine, increased blood urea, increased blood uric acid, pyrexia, asthenia, chills, and malaise.

3.4.8   Alpha Interferon

Alpha interferon 2b may increase the risk of hypersensitivity reactions such as skin redness, itching, and low blood pressure—symptoms that can be serious. Periodontal and dental disorders, altered mental status, loss of consciousness, acute hypersensitivity reactions including hives, angioedema, bronchoconstriction, and anaphylaxis have been reported, but their frequency is unknown.

Appropriating the knowledge of the potential reactions and probable complications in pregnancy submitted to chemotherapy, the professional who monitors a case of leukemia during pregnancy is partly aware of the possible situations to be faced because the response to chemotherapy also contemplates the character individual physiological response, general health status of the pregnant woman, covering important points such as nutrition, hydration, and psychological health, among other interfering issues. Thus, as already mentioned in this chapter, the delay in starting treatment can also have severe consequences for both mother and fetus.

In this sense and to demonstrate in practical terms, a study that sought to report the outcomes resulting from the clinical management/treatment for acute leukemia in 23 pregnant women concluded that about 50% of pregnant women diagnosed with acute leukemia in the second and third trimester (who delayed chemotherapy treatment for more than a week) died when they started receiving induction therapy, during this treatment. The 11 patients who received chemotherapy during pregnancy had four fetal losses and, of seven deliveries, five were at term and two were premature. In the study, there were no reports of cases with congenital malformations. And, in 18 patients (78%), there was complete remission of the disease, but in a 55-month follow-up, seven patients remained alive—which corresponds to 30% of the total [21].

In this objective of surveying the protocols used in pregnant women with leukemia, there are the difficulties described by Shapira, Pereg, and Lishner (2008): due to the prevalence of leukemia in pregnancy being low (approximately 1–100,000), there is an impediment to perform great prospective studies, in order to bring up the problems related to the diagnosis, the clinical management of these women during pregnancy, and the results of this treatment [22].

Thus, the teratogenicity of individual chemotherapeutic agents must be interpreted with the understanding that data are limited and collected from a heterogeneous group of patients for an extended period of treatment. The mother should always be advised and be aware of the risks related to treatment and of continuing with the pregnancy, in addition to the side effects and the impact of therapy on the newborn. The effects on the fetus, not only of cytotoxic therapy but also of the additional therapy that may be used (such as antibiotics and antifungals), must be considered and even evaluated in their protocols through the gonadal function [23].

Thus, there is still a difficulty, although diminished over the years, in finding available literature for consultation of regimens of chemotherapy protocols used in pregnant women with leukemia and, when found, the vast majority are configured as case studies—often sporadic individual or a small representative portion. This shows us the need for research in the area, in order to fill the gaps still present in the treatment of pregnant women with leukemia and to promote the conduct that has good results for both the mother and the baby's future.

References

1. Gonçalves, et al. Diagnosis and treatment of cervical cancer during pregnancy. Sao Paulo Med J. 2009;127(6):359.
2. Fernandes, et al. Prognosis of breast cancer in pregnancy: evidence for nursing care. Lat Am J Nurs. 2011;19(6):1453.
3. Nomura RMY, et al. Maternal and perinatal outcomes in pregnant women with leukemia. Braz J Gynecol Obstet. 2011;33(8):174.
4. Fonseca AJ, et al. Neoadjuvant chemotherapy followed by radical surgery in a pregnant patient with cervical cancer: case report and literature review. Braz J Gynecol Obstet. 2011;33(1):43.
5. Ali S, et al. Guidelines for the diagnosis and management of acute myeloid leukaemia in pregnancy. Br J Haematol. 2015;170:487–95.
6. Chelghoum Y, Vey N, Raffoux E, Huguet F, Pigneux A, Witz B, et al. Acute leukemia during pregnancy: a report on 37 patients and a review of the literature. Cancer. 2005;104(1):110–7.
7. Kebriaei P, Champlin R, Lima M, Estey E. Management of Acute Leukemias. In: de Vita Jr VT, et al., editors. Cancer: principles practice of oncology. 9th ed. Philadelphia: Lippincott Williams&Wilkins; 2011. Chap. 131. p. 1928–54.
8. Chauffaille MLLF. Acute Myelocytic leukemia. Chap. 165. In: Lopes AC, et al., editors. Medical clinic treaty., Ed. Roca; 2006. p. 2026–39.
9. Szer J. The prevelant predicament of relapsed acute myeloid leukemia. In: HEMATOLOGY American Society of Hematology education program book, vol. 1(43); 2012. p. 42–8.
10. Vardiman JW, Brunning RD, Arber DA, et al. Introduction and overview of the classification of the myeloid neoplasm. Chap.1. In: Swerdlow SH, et al., editors. WHO classification of tumours of haematopoietic and lymphoid tissues. 4th ed. Lyon: Intern. Agency for Research on Cancer/IARC Press; 2008. p. 18–30.
11. Lopes A, Lyeyasu H, Castro RMRPS. Oncology for graduation. 2nd ed. Sao Paulo: Tecmedd; 2008.
12. Sanz MA, et al. Management of acute promyelocytic leukemia: recommendations from an expert panel on behalf of the European LeukemiaNet. Blood. 2009;113(9):1875.
13. Homrich SS. Nanocapsules containing all-trans-retinoic acid: antitumor effect via cell differentiation and intrinsic apoptotic activation in acute promyelocytic leukemia cells [Dissertation]. Santa Maria, RS: Franciscan University Center of Santa Maria; 2017.
14. Gurney JG, Severson RK, Davis S, Robison LL. Incidence of cancer in children in the United States. Sex- race and 1-year age-specific rates by histologic type. Cancer. 1995;75:2186–95.
15. Pui CH. Acute lymphoblastic leukemia. Pediatr Clin N Am. 1997;44:831–46.
16. Brenner MK, Pinkel D. Cure of leukemia. Semin Hematol. 1999;36:73–83.

17. Pedrosa F, Lins M. Acute lymphoid leukemia: a curable disease. Braz J Mater Child Health. 2002;2:1.
18. Döhner H, Estey EH, Amadori S, et al. Diagnosis and management of acute myeloid leukemia in adults: recommendations from an international expert panel, on behalf of the European LeukemiaNet. Blood. 2010;115:453–74.
19. Ministry of Health (BR). Ordinance No. 649, of November 11, 2008. Therapeutic guidelines for adult chronic myeloid leukemia. Health Care Secretariat. Brasília, DF. Available in: http://bvsms.saude.gov.br/bvs/saudelegis/sas/2008/prt0649_11_11_2008.html. Accessed on 18 Feb 2020.
20. Huifang Z, Yongping S, Zhen L, et al. Effects of nilotinib exposure on pregnancy outcome in patients with chronic myeloid leukemia [J]. Chin J Hematol. 2019;40(12):986–9. https://doi.org/10.3760/cma.j.issn.0253-2727.2019.12.003.
21. Farhadfar N, Cerquozzi S, Hessenauer MR, Litzow MR, Hogan WJ, Letendre L, Patnaik MM, Tefferi A, Gangat N. Acute leukemia in pregnancy: a single institution experience with 23 patients. Leuk Lymphoma. 2017;58(5):1052–60. https://doi.org/10.1080/10428194.2016.1222379.
22. Shapira T, Pereg D, Lishner M. How I treat acute and chronic leukemia in pregnancy. 5th ed. Boold Rev. 2008;22:247–59.
23. Milojkovic D, Apperley JF. How I treat leukemia during pregnancy4th ed. Blood. 2014;123(7):974–84.
24. Thomas DA, et al. Chemoimmunotherapy with a modified hyper-CVAD and rituximab regimen improves outcome in De Novo Philadelphia chromosome–negative precursor B-lineage acute lymphoblastic leukemia. J Clin Oncol. 2010;28:3880–9.
25. Namura RMY, et al. Resultados maternos e perinatais em gestantes portadoras de leucemia. Rev. Bras. Ginecol. Obstet. 33(8). Rio de Janeiro. Aug. 2011.

Chapter 4
Pharmacokinetics and Pharmacodynamics of Chemotherapy for Leukemia in Pregnancy

William Rotea Jr.

4.1 Introduction

Despite the risks that a drug may present to a developing fetus, several types of medications can be prescribed to pregnant women, most times without any specific validation of the effects in this population. Reasons to use a drug therapy during gestation include cases of preexisting chronic diseases (i.e., asthma, hypertension, and diabetes mellitus, among many others) or for the treatment of incident conditions, which can be pregnancy-related complications or newly developed illnesses, among them, a malignant disease [4].

Introducing a treatment during pregnancy may turn into a challenging situation to prescribers and patients, as this underlying condition induces several changes on the physiology that may change the pharmacokinetics (PK) and pharmacodynamics of drugs. Changing the pharmacological behavior of a medication in the body may affect the efficacy of the therapy, and there is also the possibility of unwanted effects of these drugs on the patient and the fetus. Pregnant women are not usually included in clinical trials; therefore, most of our knowledge of drug utilization in this population are from in vitro studies, animal models, and observational or retrospective reports.

Pregnancy-related cancer can be defined as a diagnosis of a malignancy occurring 3 months before an abortion, 9 months before a delivery, or within 12 months after the pregnancy outcome [19]. It is a relatively uncommon event, with an overall incidence between 0.1% and 0.2% of all pregnancies, but this figure is expected to increase, as women are opting for conception at later age [9, 5, 16, 43]. The incidence of specific types of tumor may vary in different populations, depending also on the period evaluated; however, most frequently reported tumors are breast, melanoma, cervix, and

W. Rotea Jr. (✉)
Oncology Pharmacist, São Paulo, Brazil

© Springer Nature Switzerland AG 2021
C. W. P. Schmidt, K. M. Otoni (eds.), *Chemotherapy and Pharmacology for Leukemia in Pregnancy*, https://doi.org/10.1007/978-3-030-54058-6_4

Table 4.1 Incidence of cancers during pregnancy: case series and common types

Location	Finland	Australia	USA	Japan	Italy
Years	1950–1969	1994–2008	2001–2013	2014	2003–2015
Pregnancies	153,424	1,309,501	775,709	215,372	682,173
Malignancies	87	499	846	189	867
Incidence	0.056%	0.038%	0.109%	0.09%	0.127%
Breast	28%	19%	25%	24%	30%
Melanoma	6%	40%	11%	–	5%
Cervix	20%	5%	9%	36%	3%
Thyroid/ endocrine	10%	8%	20%	4%	18%
Hematological	8%	11%	10%	10%	12%
Colorectal	–	2%	–	5%	3%

Adapted from Eastwood-Wilshere et al. [19]

hematologic malignancies, which match with the incidence of tumors during the reproductive age of women in the general population. (Table 4.1).

The incidence of hematologic malignancies in pregnancy is lower, around 0.02%. However, this group of diseases englobes several different cancers, like Hodgkin's/ non-Hodgkin's lymphomas and diverse types of leukemia. Therefore, facing a diagnosis of a specific subtype of this group of diseases may be a unique situation for health professionals. No comprehensive guidelines are available for the management of these types of cancers in pregnant women, and the treatment plan needs to be individualized. For the patients, some decisions during the therapy may potentially be influenced by personal, ethical, and social aspects. In selected cases, termination of pregnancy may be required, but in recent years, this approach has become less frequent. For most cases, there are therapeutic options that can be applied in a safe manner [29, 33, 34].

The desirable goal of therapy is to maximize the efficacy of antineoplastic agents, leading to the best outcome for the mother, without causing any impact on the development of the fetus or late effects to the child. To achieve this balance, it is important to understand the changes that occur in mother's physiology during pregnancy and seek for dosing strategies that result in an optimized pharmacotherapy to this population [18, 30, 41].

4.2 Pharmacokinetic Changes in Pregnancy

It is a premise that a drug needs to reach the target tissue at a significant concentration in order to have a pharmacological effect in the body. Pharmacokinetics (PK) describes the time course of concentration of a drug and its metabolites in compartments of the body, since its administration until elimination. PK is constituted by the following stages: drug absorption, distribution, metabolism, elimination, and transport.

In general, we may define pregnancy as a dynamic state with accelerated metabolism, increased plasma volume and body fat, reduced vascular resistance, and decreased plasma protein concentration. Enzymatic metabolism in liver may also change during gestation; some enzymes present higher activity while in others the activity is reduced. These pregnancy-induced changes in the mother's body can affect the stages of PK mentioned above, modifying the profile and dosing of some drugs, with possible impacts on efficacy and safety of the therapy.

Since these physiologic changes may be clinically relevant, further studies are needed to address the efficacy, risks, and required adjustments associated with drug therapy in the specific context of pregnancy. If the changes in PK profile of the drug lead to lower concentrations of the drug in the target tissue, the efficacy of the therapy decreases and the fetus will be unnecessarily exposed to a potential risk. On the other hand, elevated concentrations of the drug may increase the risk of toxicity.

4.2.1 Absorption

Absorption is the passage of a drug from the site of administration into systemic circulation. This process is intrinsically related to "bioavailability," which is a fraction of an active drug that reaches the systemic circulation. Intravascular administration delivers the drug directly into the blood; no absorption occurs by this route and bioavailability is 100%. Pharmacokinetic profile of some drugs administered by intramuscular and subcutaneous routes can be influenced by changes in the blood flow at the site of administration (i.e., vasodilatation, exercise, etc.) and by characteristics of the drug (i.e., physical properties, formulation, etc.), but no pregnancy-related factor is known to affect these routes [20].

The most variable route on bioavailability is oral administration. Several circumstances can potentially affect the amount of drug that effectively reaches the blood stream. Gastric acid production is lower in pregnancy and mucus secretion is higher, leading to an elevation of pH in the stomach. This can be particularly important when the drug is a weak acid, as the increased ionization at high pH values may reduce the absorption. Weak bases, on the other hand, would predominantly stay unionized, favoring absorption. Pregnancy is also associated with nausea and vomiting, mainly in the first trimester, which may eliminate a significant part of the administered drug from the body. Other possible implicated factors in oral route are concomitant food intake, increased gut transit time, gut metabolism, uptake, and efflux transport.

Despite the potential disturbances in absorption, no published data confirm the influence any of the above factors in drug therapy during pregnancy. Studies with β-adrenoreceptor antagonist and β-lactam antibacterials comparing oral and intravenous routes on late pregnancy and postpartum showed no difference in bioavailability between these periods. Therefore, it seems that pregnancy-related gastrointestinal changes may have less impact on the bioavailability of drugs. Other pregnancy changes, like increase cardiac output and intestinal blood flow, may balance the reduced absorption [4].

4.2.2 Distribution

After reaching the systemic circulation, the drug is delivered to other fluids and tissues in organs throughout the body. Each organ may present different concentrations of the drug; therefore, the concept of compartmentalization of the organism was used to describe the distribution process. In this way, distribution can be defined as a reversible transfer of a dose of medication from one location to another. The extension of distribution of a drug throughout the body is expressed by volume of distribution (V_d), which is a theoretical volume in which an administered dose of a drug would occupy if uniformly distributed at the same concentration seen in plasma. Factors that influence V_d are blood flow in the organ, perfusion rate of the tissue, and vascular permeability. Drug-related factors are lipid solubility, extension of plasma protein, and tissue binding. Drugs with a high molecular weight or highly bound to plasma proteins have a small V_d, whereas drugs that remain with a small proportion in the intravascular space or highly bound to tissues have a high V_d. V_d is a PK parameter that determines the loading dose required to achieve the desired therapeutic concentration. Changes in V_d affect peak and trough drug concentration at steady state and maximum drug concentration after a single intravenous bolus administration.

Some pregnancy-related changes may interfere with drug distribution. Among cardiac changes, there is the increase in cardiac output, which starts at the beginning of pregnancy. It reaches a plateau of around 7 L/min by 16 weeks and remains high until delivery. An increase in stroke volume also occurs by 20 weeks of gestation, and heart rate reaches 90 beats per min at rest in the third trimester. However, little information is available on the effect of pregnancy-related increase in cardiac output on hepatic blood flow, as most studies were underpowered to evaluate this question. In contrast, an increase in renal flow is observed, which affects renal filtration, creatinine clearance, and renal drug clearance.

A marked increase in total body water, plasma volume, and all body fluid compartments is observed. The range of body weight gain is from 6 to 18 kg, and around 60% of it refers to water and 30% to fat. Around 6–8 L of water is added to total body water, and maternal body fat expands around 4 kg. Consequently, the V_d for both hydrophilic and lipophilic drugs will be higher. The average steady state concentration does not change, but the peak is lower and trough higher.

The concentrations of plasma protein "albumin" and alpha 1-acid glycoprotein decrease significantly after the second trimester. This increases the amount of free drug in plasma, which may be clinically significant for highly protein-bound drugs and low extraction rate to liver. For drugs with a narrow therapeutic window, the reduced concentration of plasma proteins can significantly increase the area under the concentration-time curve of the unbound drug and therefore lead to an increased pharmacologic effect and risk of toxicity which may require a dose adjustment.

Finally, the fetus and the amniotic fluid may function as additional compartments for distribution of drugs, resulting in increase in V_d. Small molecules and lipophilic drugs are capable of crossing the placenta, which is favored by increase in blood flow to the uterus. [3, 15, 24].

4.2.3   Metabolism

Clearance is a relevant pharmacokinetic parameter. After absorption of a given dose and the distribution through several compartments and tissues, it is the ability of the body to eliminate the drug that will determine the amount of systemic exposure to the therapeutic agent.

Metabolism is the conversion of the chemical structure of the drug into others that favor its elimination from the body. Liver is the most important organ involved in metabolism, but for some drugs, it can also occur in intestines, blood, lung, kidneys, and placenta. Hepatic clearance of drugs is dependent on the amount of free drug, which is not protein-bound, liver blood flow, and metabolic enzymes [24].

Several metabolic enzymes are involved in drug metabolism. The reactions involved in phase I metabolism are mainly oxidation, reduction, and hydrolysis. As a result, more hydrophilic metabolites are produced. The most important family of enzymes involved in such reactions is the Cytochrome P450 (CYP). Phase II reactions are conjugation of the drug or metabolites produced in phase I with glucuronic acid, sulfate, glutathione, and amino acids. Among the enzymes involved are uridine diphosphate glucuronosyltransferase (UGT), N-acetyltransferase (NAT), sulfotransferase, and methyltransferase, among others. The enzymes of CYP are grouped into three subfamilies of specific isoenzymes: CYP1, CYP2, and CYP3. UGT has two subfamilies: UGT1 and UGT2. Observational studies suggest that pregnancy causes differential effects on the activity of these enzymes. CYP3A, CYP2D6, CYP2C9, and UGT show increased activity, while the activity of CYP1A2 and CYP2C19 is decreased (Table 4.2).

4.2.4   Transport

Some substances like cytokines, hormones, and other endogenous substrates need active transport to move through membranes and tissues. Drug transporters are the molecules that are distributed all over the body and contribute to the processes of absorption, distribution, and elimination of the drug.

Placenta connects the circulatory systems of the mother and the fetus, and most transfers across this organ are via passive diffusion. Physicochemical properties of

Table 4.2 Changes in the activity of main metabolic enzymes during pregnancy

Enzyme	Activity in pregnancy	Effect in metabolism
CYP1A2	Activity evaluated at 14–18 weeks, 24–28 weeks, and 36–40 weeks;~30–65% decrease in activity	Higher concentrations of CYP1A2 substrates; risk of toxicity
CYP2C19	Lower activity compared with postpartum period	Significant differences in extensive CYP2C9 metabolizers;no difference in CYP2C19 poor metabolizers
CYP2D6	Increased activity in a small number of subjects using metoprolol probe; ~25–50% increase compared with postpartum period using dextromethorphan	Decrease in concentrations of CYP2D6 substrates
CYP3A	Increased activity using midazolam probe at 28–32 weeks of gestation compared with 6–10 weeks in postpartum	Decrease in concentrations of CYP3A substrates; most important enzyme in drug metabolism
CYP2C9	Increased activity using phenytoin	Decrease in concentrations of CYP2C9 substrates
UGT1A4	Increased activity using lamotrigine	Decrease in concentrations of UGT1A4 substrates

Adapted from Herbert [25]

the drug like molecular weight, lipid solubility, maternal concentration, and pH at which the drug is ionized are relevant to placental transfer. However, some placental drug transporters were identified. They are responsible for selecting the substrates that can reach the fetus. Among placental drug transporters are the family of multi-drug resistance proteins (MRPs), phospho-glycoprotein (P-gp), and breast cancer resistance protein (BCRP). These efflux transporters work against the concentration gradient of the drug and play a significant role in protecting the fetus by removing harmful substances. The substrates of these proteins include chemotherapeutic agents like doxorubicin, epirubicin, and paclitaxel, as supported by in vitro studies using human and animal placenta tissue. Some supportive agents, like dopamine and serotonin antagonists, phenothiazines and steroids, in general used as antiemetics, are also substrates of these transporters and therefore can interfere with the transfer of chemotherapeutic agents, which may reach the fetal compartment. In vitro studies also showed that selective serotonin reuptake inhibitors (SSRIs), used as treatment for depression, can inhibit P-gp, and therefore the use of these agents can reduce the protection of these drug transporters to fetus [5, 22].

4.3 Principles of Chemotherapy for Leukemia in Pregnancy

In the past, that is, before 1960, the standard of care for an incident malignancy in pregnant woman was termination of pregnancy, as mother's health was the focus in this challenging situation. Nowadays, chemotherapy administration can be considered relatively safe to the fetus, if applied under certain circumstances. Several published case series of treated women show that, in the majority of the cases, pregnancies can result in normal outcomes, although the risk of malformations and other neonatal conditions still exist [30].

Choosing a therapeutic plan depends, at first, on a correct diagnosis. Most women are diagnosed late, as some symptoms may overlap with pregnancy signs, like weakness, shortness of breath, and abdominal and back pain. As an additional challenge, it is important to note that some diagnostic procedures and image methods require special precautions in this clinical setting. Bone marrow biopsy is considered safe, but the use of anesthesia should be weighed on risks and benefits in an individual approach. X-ray, as well computed tomography (CT) and fluorodeoxyglucose positron emission tomography (PET-CT) scans are not recommended due to radiation exposure and placental transfer of fluorodeoxyglucose. Magnetic resonance imaging without contrast and ultrasound are possible alternatives. Specific tumor type, stage of disease, gestational period, and patient-specific needs and beliefs are relevant for therapeutic decisions, but the treatment should be closest as possible to standard care of nonpregnant patients.

Exposure to chemotherapy in the first 14 days after conception, that is, the implantation phase, may result in a normal embryo or a miscarriage; this phenomenon is described as "all or none," depending on how many embryonic stem cells were affected by the drug. In the following phase, called "organogenesis," which occurs between weeks 2 and 8, the embryo is highly susceptible to drug-related teratogenicity. The estimated risk of malformations is 10–20% in monotherapy exposure and around 25% for combination of agents. For some organs and systems, like eyes, genitalia, hematopoietic system, and central nervous system, the susceptibility remains high during the whole gestation period. In the fetal phase, after week 8, previously formed organs grow and get mature. Although the probability of malformations is reduced, there is still a risk for intrauterine growth retardation, preterm delivery, and low birth weight.

4.3.1 Leukemia: General Considerations

The term "leukemia" comes from the Greek words *leukós* ("white") and *haîma* ("blood") and describes a heterogenic group of diseases that have in common the characteristic of abnormal proliferation of one or more cell lines in the bone marrow. Classification of leukemias is based on the type of cell, that is, myeloid or lymphoid, and the clinical course of the disease, that is, acute or chronic. Acute leukemias present rapid growth and poorly differentiated cells and chronic forms have slow progressive accumulation of cells in bone marrow and peripheral tissues. Based on these simple criteria and considering the relevance for women in reproductive age, the main types of leukemia are: acute myeloid leukemia (AML), chronic myeloid leukemia (CML), and acute lymphoblastic leukemia (ALL).

The WHO (World Health Organization) classification of hematological malig-nancies includes several other types and subtypes of the disease, as the comprehen-sive classification considers the presence of specific mutations and other genetic alterations that have impact on diagnosis and prognosis, but they are out of the scope of this chapter.

4.3.2 Acute Myeloid Leukemia

It is the most common type of acute leukemia in adults and is responsible for the largest number of deaths from the disease. The age-adjusted incidence rate of AML in general population is 3.7 cases per 100,000 men and women, and the median age of diagnosis is 66 years. The real incidence of leukemia during pregnancy is poorly defined; however, it is estimated in a range from 1 in 75,000 to 100,000 gestations. AML is the most incident type, and accounts for two-thirds of all cases. Most cases are diagnosed during the second and third trimesters of gestation. Only one out of five cases is diagnosed in the first trimester; however, the bias of underreporting due to spontaneous pregnancy termination should be considered [21].

Symptoms at diagnosis include severe anemia, thrombocytopenia, and neutrope-nia. Leukostasis, or symptomatic hyperleukocytosis, may be present and it is con-sidered an emergency, requiring leukapheresis as prompt intervention. The age of diagnosis is an important prognostic factor, as in patients ≥60 years of age there is a higher prevalence of unfavorable cytogenetic factors and comorbidities which impairs the ability to tolerate intensive treatment, which is recommended for younger subjects. The management of AML is based on chemotherapy, which is divided in two steps: induction and post-remission or consolidation. The objective of induction chemotherapy is to achieve a significant reduction in leukemic blasts and restore normal hematopoiesis. It should be introduced in the shortest period possible after diagnosis. The patient's outcome can be affected if the time of intro-duction of chemotherapy is beyond 5 days. If the diagnosis occurs in the first trimes-ter, termination of pregnancy may be recommended as the induction chemotherapy represents a high risk for the embryo. Cases diagnosed later may receive conven-tional induction regimens despite the risk of growth restriction and abortion. Soon after achievement of remission, the consolidation regimen is introduced to prevent relapse, which is expected to happen after 6–9 months without post-remission therapy.

Most regimens use a combination of cytarabine with an anthracycline, such as daunorubicin, idarubicin, or doxorubicin. Daunorubicin is preferred over the others as animal tests showed lower teratogenic potential in exposure to daunorubicin compared to doxorubicin, and it is a recommended drug in the management of AML. Idarubicin is also a valid option in this indication; however, due to a more lipophilic structure, there is the theorical increased potential to cross the placenta.

Horowitz et al. [26] published a meta-analysis of publications from January 1966 to August 2014. The authors identified 138 cases diagnosed between 1955 and

2013. From this cohort, 93 patients were treated during pregnancy, 24 were treated after abortion, and 21 after delivery. Thirty women (22%) were diagnosed in the first trimester, 74 (54%) in the second trimester, and 31 (22%) in the third trimester. Two cases were diagnosed shortly after delivery and in one case, the information was not reported. Most frequent regimens were based on combination of cytarabine with doxorubicin, idarubicin, daunorubicin, or mitoxantrone ($n = 54$, 58%). Non-anthracycline regimens were the second most frequent choice ($n = 33$, 34%), followed by steroids alone, applied as "bridging" therapy ($n = 7$, 8%). Live birth was the outcome of 89 pregnancies, 22 were elective abortions, and 23 losses. A higher proportion of infants exposed to chemotherapy had a low birth weight, but with no statistical significance in the difference. Four cases presented anomalies, described as unspecified deformations, that is, patent ductus arteriosus, hydrocephalus, and ventricular septum defect. Complete remission rate of patients treated during pregnancy was 87%, which was comparable to remission rate achieved in post-delivery-treated cohort (82%) and age-matched nonpregnant females.

Chang and Patel [12] published a systematic review of literature in which they included reports from AML treatment during pregnancy. The search found 83 women and 85 fetuses exposed to chemotherapy in the period from January 1969 to June 2014. Several chemotherapy agents were used in different regimens. Authors collected information on time of therapy introduction and mother's and baby's outcomes. They also performed an analysis of these indicators based on all the drugs reported in the publications. The results are tabulated in Tables 4.2 and 4.3.

Newborns experienced some side effects of the therapy, of which the most common side effect was anemia. The events included also myelosuppression, hepatopathy, acrocyanosis, seizures, hyaline membrane disease, respiratory distress syndrome, and infections. Chromosome abnormalities, such as Down's syndrome and inversion of chromosome 9, were reported in two cases. Four infants had growth defects. One case presented sacral dimple, short digits and limbs, and a prominent frontal skull with macrognathia. There was one case of hypospadias and one of congenital adherence of iris to posterior cornea in the left eye. The last was a case of polydactyly, which was associated to family history (Tables 4.4, 4.5, and 4.6).

Authors conclude that treatment of AML in the second and third trimesters resulted in fewer complications and less fetal loss than treatments introduced in first trimester. Complete remission rate was lower in second and third trimester treatments, which could partially be explained by a delay in the introduction of therapy, although it was considered comparable to nonpregnant patients.

Table 4.3 Outcomes of pregnancies based on the time of introduction of chemotherapy for AML

	Mothers	Spontaneous abortions – n (%)	Complete remission	Live births
1st trimester	8	3 (37.5%)	100%	5
2nd trimester	61	6 (9.7%)	81%	56
3rd trimester	14	0	67%	15

From Chang and Patel [12]

Table 4.4 Infant's and mother's outcomes based on drug used in chemotherapy for AML in first trimester

	Number of treatments 1st trimester	Infant's outcome		Mother's outcome					
		Live births	Death	CR	Relapse after CR	PR	PD/ Death	NR
Cytarabine	8	5	3	6	2	0	0	2
Daunorubicin	4	2	2	1	0	0	0	3
Doxorubicin	5	5	0	5	1	0	0	0
Vincristine	5	4	1	2	0	0	0	3

From Chang and Patel [12]
CR Complete Response, *PR* Partial Response, *PD* Progressive Disease

Table 4.5 Infant's and mother's outcomes based on drug used in chemotherapy for AML in second trimester

	Number of treatments 2nd trimester	Infant's outcome		Mother's outcome					
		Live births	Death	CR	Relapse after CR	PR	PD/ Death	NR
Cytarabine	61	56	6	43	9	2	3/5	8
Daunorubicin	38	36	3	27	0	1	3/3	4
Idarubicin	7	6	1	6	0	0	1/0	0
Doxorubicin	11	9	2	7	1	1	1/0	2
Mitoxantrone	4	2	2	3	0	0	0/1	0
Etoposide	2	2	0	2	0	0	0	0
Vincristine	5	4	1	3	0	0	0/2	0
Fludarabine	1	1	0	0	0	0	0/1	0
Cyclophosphamide	1	1	0	1	0	0	0	0

From Chang and Patel [12]
CR Complete Response, *PR* Partial Response, *PD* Progressive Disease

Table 4.6 Infant's and mother's outcomes based on drug used in chemotherapy for AML in third trimester

	Number of treatments 3rd trimester	Infant's outcome		Mother's outcome					
		Live births	Death	CR	Relapse after CR	PR	PD/ Death	NR
Cytarabine	14	15	0	7	0	3	1/0	3
Daunorubicin	6	6	0	4	0	0	1/0	1
Idarubicin	1	1	0	0	0	0	0	1
Doxorubicin	3	3	0	1	0	2	0	0
Mitoxantrone	1	1	0	1	0	0	0	0
Vincristine	5	6	0	3	0	2	0	0

From Chang and Patel [12]
CR Complete Response, *PR* Partial Response, *PD* Progressive Disease

Mabed et al. [31] published a report of a single institution series of 27 cases of acute leukemia, which included 18 diagnoses of AML. The data of these patients were matched with a group of 75 nonpregnant patients. The authors' conclusion was that pregnancy did not impact the outcome of the patients.

4.3.3 Acute Promyelocytic Leukemia

This is an invasive subtype of AML, which accounts for approximately 10% of the cases of the disease. The main genetic feature of APL is the chromosomal translocation that juxtaposes the *PML* (Promyelocytic Leukemia) gene on Chromosome 15 with the *RARα* (Retinoic Acid Receptor) gene from Chromosome 17. This translocation produces a chimeric protein PML-RARα that is found in over 95% of human APLs and causes a block on maturation of neutrophils at promyelocytic level. PML-RARα affects the function of the native PML protein, which is essential to many apoptotic pathways and is implicated in the control of genomic stability [10, 17, 38].

Clinical symptoms at diagnosis include pancytopenia, disseminated intravascular coagulation, and hyperfibrinolysis. APL has a high risk of maternal and/or fetal death, intra uterine growth restriction (IUGR), and preterm delivery. Patients may also experience bleeding, infection, inflammation, placental abruption, and decreased oxygen and nutrient supply to fetus.

Treatment for APL is carried out with exposure to all-trans retinoic acid (ATRA), as this drug induces in vivo differentiation of APL blasts. ATRA causes the degradation the PML-RARα through the ubiquitin-proteasome and caspase system after binding to retinoic acid receptors in the structure of this fusion protein. This results in restoration of terminal differentiation of promyelocytes. However, this drug cannot eliminate the leukemic clone, and therefore a combination with anthracycline-based chemotherapy is normally used. This regimen has a complete remission rate of >90% and around 80% of patients have potential cure. However, ATRA is highly teratogenic if used in first trimester, and it should be avoided. Termination of pregnancy may be considered. Anomalies include craniofacial alterations, neural tube defects, cardiovascular malformations, and thymic aplasia. If used after the second trimester, the teratogenic risk is low. One possible alternative is postponing the use of the anthracycline to post delivery and giving ATRA as a single agent. This approach is not recommended to high-risk patients with hyperleukocytosis [17, 28].

Another drug used in the therapy of PML is the arsenic trioxide (ATO). This agent degrades the PML-RARα by acting on PML moiety; however, the use of ATO cannot be recommended in any stage of pregnancy since it is extremely toxic to fetus [10].

4.3.4 Acute Lymphoblastic Leukemia

Acute lymphoblastic leukemia is caused by the proliferation and accumulation of lymphoid progenitor cells in bone marrow and adjacent tissues. The age-adjusted incidence rate of ALL in general population is 1.7 cases per 100,000. Around 60%

of cases occur before 20 years of age and higher incidence of the remaining cases is in the fifth decade of life. In pregnancy, ALL corresponds to a little less than one-third of all leukemias.

Treatment of ALL in adults does not have the same results as that in children. The estimated cure rate is 20–40% against 80% in pediatric population. Adults have higher risk features, higher relapse rates after complete remission, and predisposition to resistance to chemotherapy [27].

Combination regimens of agents are recommended after week 20 of gestation; before that period, elective termination of pregnancy may be considered. Alternatively, 1–2 weeks of treatment with prednisolone may be considered until the patient enters week 20 and resumes chemotherapy. Use of methotrexate is not recommended before the third trimester; hence, the approach with steroids can also be used for the patient enter in this period and, if necessary, receive this therapy. Most common chemotherapeutic agents used in this malignancy are doxorubicin, cyclophosphamide and vincristine (in the hyperfractionated CVAD regimen). Other combinations include asparaginase and vincristine, together with steroids and anthracyclines. Asparaginase may increase the risk of thromboembolic events, which is already high due to the combination of pregnancy and malignancy [40].

In a series of 17 patients with ALL, reported by Terek et al. [39], about half of the patients achieved remission while the same amount relapsed or had fatal disease progression; treatment was given between 15 and 33 weeks and most patients received anthracyclines, vincristine and steroids. Perinatal complications included transient pancytopenia, respiratory distress and preterm delivery.

One important cytogenetic abnormality in ALL is Philadelphia chromosome (Ph), affecting around 20–30% of cases. Ph results from a reciprocal translocation between the ABL-1 oncogene on the long arm of chromosome 9 and a breakpoint cluster region (BCR) on the long arm of chromosome 22. The fusion gene, BCR-ABL, encodes an oncogenic protein with constitutively active tyrosine kinase activity. Ph-positive ALL have a poor prognostic with traditional chemotherapy, therefore tyrosine kinase inhibitors (TKI), targeting BCR-ABL protein, were introduced in the management of disease. First in class was Imatinib, followed by second and third generation agents nilotinib, dasatinib, bosutinib and ponatinib, developed mainly for imatinib-resistant patients. These agents showed teratogenicity in animal models and should be used with caution, out of organogenesis phase of pregnancy.

4.3.5 Chronic Myeloid Leukemia

The reciprocal translocation between the chromosomes 9 and 22 is the cornerstone in the clinical development of CML, and the test for this cytogenetic feature is sensitive for the confirmation of the diagnosis, as the Ph is detected in around 90% of the cases. This oncogene activates multiple transduction pathways that induce growth, proliferation, and changes in cellular adhesion and inhibit apoptosis of early hematopoietic progenitor cells. The incidence rate of CML in general population is 1.8

cases per 100,000, and the frequency is higher among males than females. The median age of diagnosis is 55–60 years, and only 17% of cases occur between 20 and 44 years of age. In pregnancy, CML corresponds to less than 1 in 10,000 pregnancies [8, 13, 32, 35].

Introduction of TKIs in the treatment of CML changed the prognosis and survival of the patients dramatically. In most cases, long-lasting responses and high tolerability of therapy are observed. TKIs are designed to compete with adenosine triphosphate (ATP) to bind to the catalytic site of BCR-ABL protein. In this way, when ATP is prevented from reaching the enzyme, the phosphorylation process is blocked and the signaling pathways that promote leukemogenesis are switched off. Animal tests with TKIs demonstrated teratogenicity of the agents and less extent of effect in fertility; therefore, the exposure to these agents may result in serious fetal malformations [2].

Pye et al. [36] published a large series of 180 cases of imatinib exposure during pregnancy. Four women were treated for gastrointestinal stromal tumors (GISTs), 28 for unknown indications, and 5 for miscellaneous conditions. One hundred and three patients started therapy in first trimester, 4 started after that period, and 38 received therapy throughout pregnancy. Timing of exposure was unknown in 34 cases and 1 patient had started the therapy before getting pregnant. Outcome of pregnancy was unknown in 55 cases; losses occurred in 54 cases: 18 cases of spontaneous abortion; 35 cases of elective termination of gestation and 1 case of stillbirth. In 63 pregnancies, the outcome was live birth without any anomaly. In total, defects were observed in 12 fetuses: in the stillbirth case, in 3 of the elective terminations, and 8 infants were born with anomalies. In 10 of these cases, the exposure was in first trimester and in the 2 remaining cases, the time of exposure is unknown. Bone malformations and renal, respiratory, and gastrointestinal anomalies were observed. The proposed mechanism of these congenital anomalies was inhibition of tyrosine kinases; many of them are involved in embryogenic development and angiogenesis, which could affect placental circulation and nutrient distribution to fetus. Abruzzese et al. [1] added 54 pregnancies to this series, and among these cases, 5 were of congenital anomalies in infants with exposure to imatinib in first trimester. The anomalies in both reports were similar to the ones observed in animal preclinical studies, which reinforces the role of the drug in these events.

There are other case series reporting the exposure to nilotinib and dasatinib, according to Abruzzese et al. [1]. With respect to nilotinib, 50 pregnancies and 5 anomalies were registered, including a case of twins in which 1 died and other had a nonserious heart murmur.

Cortes et al. [14] published a report of 46 pregnancies with exposure to dasatinib. Twenty-six terminations of gestation occurred, of which 18 were elective and 8 spontaneous. Ten cases had anomalies identified, of which five were among the early termination group.

These molecular agents have promoted long-lasting responses with high quality of life for patients. In this scenario, despite the teratogenic potential of the therapy, for some selected patients conception may be possible. Patients in molecular response may interrupt the therapy just before or immediately after conception and return to the therapy after delivery. Since interruption of therapy is not recommended in nonpregnant population, careful planning and close supervision are required for this approach [2, 32].

4.4 Considerations for Use of Chemotherapy

Despite the limitations in design and conduction of studies evaluating the use of chemotherapeutic drugs in pregnancy, some groups have published objective results from studies. Through this growing experience, it is expected that health professionals feel more confident to treat the patients under this condition.

Van Calsteren K et al. [41] outlined some important points for establishing a therapeutic plan. Selected agents have demonstrated to be safe for the fetus. Chemotherapy can be considered between 14 and 35 weeks' gestation, a period in which the risk of teratogenic events is reduced, as confirmed by short-term outcome studies which did not show an increase in congenital malformations. On the other hand, other perinatal complications like preterm delivery, intrauterine growth restriction, hematopoietic suppression, and stillbirth have an increased risk.

Avilés, Neri and Nambo, [6, 7] and Han et al. [23] reported results from a long-term follow-up of 54 newborns exposed to chemotherapy for hematological malignancies (14 leukemia patients) in the first trimester of pregnancy (median follow-up – 22.4 years; range – 3.8–32.0 years). Chemotherapy was used at regular doses. Most frequent finding was low birth weight. Patients in this series had no abnormalities and their physical, psychological, and neurological developments were normal. No long-term events in cardiac function or neoplasms were detected.

Amant et al. [3] pointed that dose calculations, which for most drugs are based on body surface area, may not be adequate to pregnant women. Increase in plasma volume and cardiac output leading to increase in volume of distribution and glomerular filtration result in reduced plasma concentration. This hypothesis was confirmed for doxorubicin, epirubicin, carboplatin, and paclitaxel, which showed decreased AUC (Area Under the Curve) in a concentration-time plot. This implies a reduced exposure to the agent and possibly an underestimated dose. However, the clinical significance of this fact is yet to be determined as some reports have shown a comparable efficacy of therapy with nonpregnant population.

Ryu et al. [37] evaluated the PK of doxorubicin during pregnancy compared to previously published data from nonpregnant subjects. A significant decrease in clearance was observed with no changes in other parameters. Therefore, no strategy for dose adjustment was recommended.

Van Hasselt JG et al. [42] evaluated gestational effects on PK parameters of four drugs in comparison to nonpregnant controls. They observed a decrease of 5.3%, 8.2%, 14.5%, and 27.4% in the AUC of doxorubicin, epirubicin, docetaxel, and paclitaxel, respectively. These results do not support the approach of dose reductions as a protective measure as it may have an impact on the efficacy of therapy and the fetus would be unnecessarily exposed to a suboptimal treatment.

Burwick et al. [11] published a report of measurements of imatinib levels in maternal blood, placental tissue, amniotic fluid, umbilical cord blood, breast milk, and neonatal urine. The drug was administered at 28 weeks of gestation and the patient had complete hematological response within 4 weeks. No significant maternal or neonatal adverse effects were noted, but imatinib and, the main metabolite, N-desmethyl imatinib were detected in breastmilk and neonatal urine.

References

1. Abruzzese E, Trawinska MM, de Fabritiis P, Baccarani M. Management of pregnant chronic myeloid leukemia patients. Expert Rev Hematol. 2016;9:781–91. https://doi.org/10.1080/17474086.2016.
2. Abruzzese E, Trawinska MM, Perrotti AP, De Fabritiis P. Tyrosine kinase inhibitors and pregnancy. Mediterr J Hematol Infect Dis. 2014;6:e2014028. https://doi.org/10.4084/MJHID.2014.028.
3. Amant F, Han SN, Gziri MM, Dekrem J, Van Calsteren K. Chemotherapy during pregnancy. Curr Opin Oncol. 2012;24:580–6. https://doi.org/10.1097/CCO.0b013e328354e754.
4. Anderson GD. Pregnancy-induced changes in pharmacokinetics: a mechanistic-based approach. Clin Pharmacokinet. 2005;44:989–1008. https://doi.org/10.2165/00003088-200544100-00001.
5. Autio K, Rassnick KM, Bedford-Guaus SJ. Chemotherapy during pregnancy: a review of the literature. Vet Comp Oncol. 2007;5:61–75. https://doi.org/10.1111/j.1476-5829.2006.00119.x.
6. Avilés A, Neri N, Nambo MJ. Author's reply: chemotherapy during first trimester of pregnancy. Int J Cancer. 2013;132:1729. https://doi.org/10.1002/ijc.27818.
7. Avilés A, Neri N, Nambo MJ. Hematological malignancies and pregnancy: treat or no treat during first trimester. Int J Cancer. 2012;131:2678–83. https://doi.org/10.1002/ijc.27560.
8. Barkoulas T, Hall PD. Experience with dasatinib and nilotinib use in pregnancy. J Oncol Pharm Pract. 2018;24:121–8. https://doi.org/10.1177/1078155217692399.
9. Barzilai M, Avivi I, Amit O. Hematological malignancies during pregnancy. Mol Clin Oncol. 2019;10:3–9. https://doi.org/10.3892/mco.2018.1759.
10. Bassi SC, Rego EM. Molecular basis for the diagnosis and treatment of acute promyelocytic leukemia. Rev Bras Hematol Hemoter. 2012;34:134–9. https://doi.org/10.5581/1516-8484.20120033.
11. Burwick RM, Kuo K, Brewer D, Druker BJ. Maternal, fetal, and neonatal Imatinib levels with treatment of chronic myeloid leukemia in pregnancy. Obstet Gynecol. 2017;129:831–4. https://doi.org/10.1097/AOG.0000000000001972.
12. Chang A, Patel S. Treatment of acute myeloid leukemia during pregnancy. Ann Pharmacother. 2015;49:48–68. https://doi.org/10.1177/1060028014552516.
13. Chauffaille Mde L, Almeida AC, Martinez RM, Silva ASG. Frequency and diversity of variant Philadelphia chromosome in chronic myeloid leukemia patients. Blood. 2011;118:4903. https://doi.org/10.1182/blood.V118.21.4903.4903.
14. Cortes JE, Abruzzese E, Chelysheva E, Guha M, Wallis N, Apperley JF. The impact of dasatinib on pregnancy outcomes. Am J Hematol. 2015;90:1111–5. https://doi.org/10.1002/ajh.24186.
15. Costantine MM. Physiologic and pharmacokinetic changes in pregnancy. Front Pharmacol. 2014;5:65. https://doi.org/10.3389/fphar.2014.00065.
16. Danet C, Araujo M, Bos-Thompson MA, Portolan G, Gautier S, Vanlemmens L, Bonenfant S, Jonville-Béra AP, Cottin J, Vial T, Bavoux F, Montastruc JL, Damase-Michel C, Benevent J, Bourgeois-Mondon I, Lacroix I. Pregnancy outcomes in women exposed to cancer chemotherapy. Pharmacoepidemiol Drug Saf. 2018;27:1302–8. https://doi.org/10.1002/pds.4689.

17. Degos L, Wang ZY. All trans retinoic acid in acute promyelocytic leukemia. Oncogene. 2001;20:7140–5. https://doi.org/10.1038/sj.onc.1204763.
18. Dekrem J, Van Calsteren K, Amant F. Effects of fetal exposure to maternal chemotherapy. Paediatr Drugs. 2013;15:329–34. https://doi.org/10.1007/s40272-013-0040-6.
19. Eastwood-Wilshere N, Turner J, Oliveira N, Morton A. Cancer in pregnancy. Asia Pac J Clin Oncol. 2019;15:296–308. https://doi.org/10.1111/ajco.13235.
20. Feghali M, Venkataramanan R, Caritis S. Pharmacokinetics of drugs in pregnancy. Semin Perinatol. 2015;39:512–9. https://doi.org/10.1053/j.semperi.2015.08.003.
21. Fracchiolla NS, Sciumè M, Dambrosi F, Guidotti F, Ossola MW, Chidini G, Gianelli U, Merlo D, Cortelezzi A. Acute myeloid leukemia and pregnancy: clinical experience from a single center and a review of the literature. BMC Cancer. 2017;17:442. https://doi.org/10.1186/s12885-017-3436-9.
22. Framarino-Dei-Malatesta M, Sammartino P, Napoli A. Does anthracycline-based chemotherapy in pregnant women with cancer offer safe cardiac and neurodevelopmental outcomes for the developing fetus? BMC Cancer. 2017;17:777. https://doi.org/10.1186/s12885-017-3772-9.
23. Han SN, Gziri MM, Van Calsteren K, Amant F. Is chemotherapy during the first trimester of pregnancy really safe? Int J Cancer. 2013;132:1728. https://doi.org/10.1002/ijc.27815.
24. Hebert M. Impact of pregnancy on maternal pharmacokinetics of medications. In: Mattison DR, editor. Clinical pharmacology during pregnancy: Academic Press; 2013. p. 17–39. https://doi.org/10.1016/B978-0-12-386007-1.00003-9.
25. Hebert M. Impact of pregnancy on pharmacokinetics of medications. J Popul Ther Clin Pharmacol. 2013;20(3):e350–7.
26. Horowitz NA, Henig I, Henig O, Benyamini N, Vidal L, Avivi I. Acute myeloid leukemia during pregnancy: a systematic review and meta-analysis. Leuk Lymphoma. 2018;59:610–6. https://doi.org/10.1080/10428194.2017.1347651.
27. Jabbour E, O'Brien S, Konopleva M, Kantarjian H. New insights into the pathophysiology and therapy of adult acute lymphoblastic leukemia. Cancer. 2015;121:2517–28. https://doi.org/10.1002/cncr.29383.
28. Li H, Han C, Li K, Li J, Wang Y, Xue F. New onset acute promyelocytic leukemia during pregnancy: report of 2 cases. Cancer Biol Ther. 2019;20:397–401. https://doi.org/10.1080/15384047.2018.1529122.
29. Lishner M, Avivi I, Apperley JF, Dierickx D, Evens AM, Fumagalli M, Nulman I, Oduncu FS, Peccatori FA, Robinson S, Van Calsteren K, Vandenbroucke T, Van den Heuvel F, Amant F. Hematologic malignancies in pregnancy: management guidelines from an international consensus meeting. J Clin Oncol. 2016;34:501–8. https://doi.org/10.1200/JCO.2015.62.4445.
30. Lynch CD, MJN L, Del Priore G. Chemotherapy in pregnancy. In: Mattison DR, editor. Clinical pharmacology during pregnancy: Academic Press; 2013. p. 201–15. https://doi.org/10.1016/B978-0-12-386007-1.00014-3.
31. Mabed M, Eisa N, El-Ashwah S, Talaab M. Pregnancy associated acute leukemia: single center experience. Cancer Treat Res Commun. 2018;16:53–8. https://doi.org/10.1016/j.ctarc.2018.06.002. Epub 2018 Jul 3
32. Madabhavi I, Sarkar M, Modi M, Kadakol N. Pregnancy outcomes in chronic myeloid leukemia: a single center experience. J Glob Oncol. 2019;(5):1–11. https://doi.org/10.1200/JGO.18.00211.
33. Mahmoud HK, Samra MA, Fathy GM. Hematologic malignancies during pregnancy: a review. J Adv Res. 2016;7:589–96. https://doi.org/10.1016/j.jare.2016.02.001.
34. McCormick A, Peterson E. Cancer in pregnancy. Obstet Gynecol Clin N Am. 2018;45:187–200. https://doi.org/10.1016/j.ogc.2018.01.009.
35. Moura AC, Delamain MT, Duarte GBO, Lorand-Metze I, Souza CA, Pagnano KBB. Management of chronic myeloid leukemia during pregnancy: a retrospective analysis at a single center. Hematol Transfus Cell Ther. 2019;41:125–8. https://doi.org/10.1016/j.htct.2018.10.001.

36. Pye SM, Cortes J, Ault P, Hatfield A, Kantarjian H, Pilot R, Rosti G, Apperley JF. The effects of imatinib on pregnancy outcome. Blood. 2008;111:5505–8. https://doi.org/10.1182/blood-2007-10-114900.

37. Ryu RJ, Eyal S, Kaplan HG, Akbarzadeh A, Hays K, Puhl K, Easterling TR, Berg SL, Scorsone KA, Feldman EM, Umans JG, Miodovnik M, Hebert MF. Pharmacokinetics of doxorubicin in pregnant women. Cancer Chemother Pharmacol. 2014;73:789–97. https://doi.org/10.1007/s00280-014-2406-z.

38. Saeed S, Logie C, Stunnenberg HG, Martens JH. Genome-wide functions of PML–RAR in acute promyelocytic leukaemia. Br J Cancer. 2011;104:554–8. https://doi.org/10.1038/sj.bjc.6606095.

39. Terek MC, Ozkinay E, Zekioglu O, Erhan Y, Cagirgan S, Pehlivan M, Mgoyi L. Acute leukemia in pregnancy with ovarian metastasis: a case report and review of the literature. Int J Gynecol Cancer. 2003;13:904–8.

40. Ticku J, Oberoi S, Friend S, Busowski J, Langenstroer M, Baidas S. Acute lymphoblastic leukemia in pregnancy: a case report with literature review. Ther Adv Hematol. 2013;4:313–9. https://doi.org/10.1177/2040620713492933.

41. Van Calsteren K, Amant F. Cancer during pregnancy. Acta Obstet Gynecol Scand. 2014;93:443–6. https://doi.org/10.1111/aogs.12380.

42. van Hasselt JG, van Calsteren K, Heyns L, Han S, Mhallem Gziri M, Schellens JH, Beijnen JH, Huitema AD, Amant F. Optimizing anti-cancer drug treatment in pregnant cancer patients: pharmacokinetic analysis of gestation-induced changes for doxorubicin, epirubicin, docetaxel and paclitaxel. Ann Oncol. 2014;25:2059–65. https://doi.org/10.1093/annonc/mdu140.

43. Zimran E, Hoffman R, Kremyanskaya M. Current approaches to challenging scenarios in Myeloproliferative neoplasms. Expert Rev Anticancer Ther. 2018;18:567–78. https://doi.org/10.1080/14737140.2018.1457441.

Chapter 5
Clinical Care of the Fetus and the Mother: Obstetrics Management for Patients on Treatment for Leukemia

Gilmar de Souza Osmundo Junior, Ana Maria Kondo Igai, and Rossana Pulcineli Vieira Francisco

Pregnancy is a particular moment in women's life, in which there is an overlapping of physiological, psychological, epidemiological, and social modifications of the mother. The care of clinical diseases in pregnant women should always balance the risks and benefits of medical interventions to the mother and to the fetus.

Cancer is a rare event among pregnant women, yet its diagnosis is frequently associated to the burden of several dilemmas, involving the patient, the partner, and the health team [1]. Among the malignant neoplasms, leukemias are even more uncommon, with an incidence of approximately 1 in 100,000 pregnancies [2].

There is a paucity of available literature on the management of pregnant women with leukemia. Most of the current information on the subject is obtained from retrospective studies with small samples and case reports [3]. Counselling of the pregnant woman with leukemia should always include a multidisciplinary team, consisting of oncologists, obstetricians trained on maternal-fetal medicine, neonatologists, and psychologists. It is pivotal to include a clear discussion of the maternal risks due to the leukemia versus the potential known risks to the fetus and unknown long-term risks to the child [4].

5.1 Pregnancy-Related Hematologic Changes

Pregnancy leads to deep adaptation of the maternal physiology. Such changes might result in symptoms and in modifications of common laboratory test results. Health professionals in charge of pregnant women should be familiar to the

G. de Souza Osmundo Junior (✉) · A. M. K. Igai · R. P. V. Francisco
Hospital das Clínicas, University of São Paulo, São Paulo, Brazil
e-mail: gilmar.junior@hc.fm.usp.br; ana.kondo@hc.fm.usp.br;
rossana.francisco@hc.fm.usp.br

© Springer Nature Switzerland AG 2021
C. W. P. Schmidt, K. M. Otoni (eds.), *Chemotherapy and Pharmacology for Leukemia in Pregnancy*, https://doi.org/10.1007/978-3-030-54058-6_5

pregnancy-related physiological changes, in order to prevent underestimation of maternal symptoms, misinterpretations of test results, and misdiagnosis.

Pregnancy results in a progressive increase of plasma volume since the first trimester, culminating in a total increase by approximately 50% at the third trimester [5]. This hypervolemia leads to plasmatic dilution and cardiovascular overload.

Red blood cell production is also increased during gestation, but not as markedly as the plasmatic volume expansion. Hence, there is a physiological dilutional anemia in normal pregnancies.

The World Health Organization defines the diagnosis of anemia in pregnancy by the hemoglobin threshold of 11 g/dL in the first and third trimester, and 10.5 g/dL in the second trimester [6]. Every pregnant woman must also receive an oral supplementation of iron and folic acid, in order to prevent anemia [6].

There is an increase of the white blood cell production during pregnancy and labor, which results in an increase of the white blood cell (WBC) counts and even in the sporadic finding of small counts of myelocytes and metamyelocytes in peripheral blood smear [7]. There is no standardized WBC normal value range in pregnancy, but a recent retrospective study including 1000 pregnant women has described a WBC range of $5–13 \times 10^9$/L during pregnancy and a further increase of WBC during labor ($5.3–25.3 \times 10^9$/L) [8]. Detection of blasts in peripheral blood analysis should never be attributed to the pregnancy-related changes and should always be considered a pathological finding.

Platelet counts are slightly decreased but still within the normal range ($150–450 \times 10^9$/L) in pregnancy due to plasmatic dilution and possibly to an increase of the platelet clearance. Gestational thrombocytopenia (GT) occurs in 5–11% of third-trimester pregnancies, and it is defined as a platelet count below 150×10^9/L [9]. GT is a totally benign entity, and it is usually related to neither abnormal bleeding nor severe thrombocytopenia ($<70 \times 10^9$/L) [9]. Differential diagnosis of isolated platelet counts below 100×10^9/L should include immune thrombocytopenia; hemolysis, elevated liver enzymes, and low platelets in patients with severe hypertension (HELLP) syndrome; antiphospholipid syndrome; thrombotic thrombocytopenic purpura; and other causes [9].

Hence, healthy pregnant women may present with mild manifestations such as dyspnea, malaise, anemia, and thrombocytopenia. The diagnosis of very early acute leukemias may be challenging during gestation. It is important to highlight that persistent symptoms and moderate or severe laboratory abnormalities cannot be attributed to pregnancy; thus, these cases should always prompt a thorough clinical investigation.

5.2 Maternal-Fetal Outcomes in Pregnancies Complicated by Leukemia

The perinatal outcomes of leukemia in pregnancy depend mainly on the gestational age at the diagnosis and disease type, whether it is an acute, chronic, or accelerated-phase leukemia.

Acute leukemias are severe and life-threatening medical situations in pregnancy. Non-treated acute leukemias will result in maternal death in weeks to few months [2, 10]. Pregnant women with leukemia also present higher risks of neutropenia, sepsis, post-partum hemorrhage, and venous thromboembolism (VTE) [2].

Pregnancies complicated by acute leukemia have higher incidences of miscarriage, stillbirth, and neonatal death [2, 11, 12]. Possible causes of fetal death are maternal severe anemia, intravascular disseminated coagulation, and the occlusion of placental vessels by leukemic cells. Placental metastasis and mother-to-child transmission of the leukemia have also been described, but they are extremely rare events [13, 14].

The effects of fetal exposure to maternal chemotherapy depend on the type of drugs and gestational age. In general, exposition to chemotherapy in the first trimester increases the odds of miscarriage and stillbirth. It is also associated with a diverse range of congenital anomalies [3, 15, 16].

Pregnant women on chemotherapy during second and third trimester may develop intrauterine growth restriction, preterm delivery, and low-birth-weight newborns in approximately half of the cases [2, 3, 11, 12]. Stillbirth and severe placental insufficiency with abnormal umbilical artery doppler have been described in a series of case reports of leukemia during pregnancy [12].

Moreover, fetal exposure to maternal chemotherapy may increase the risks of fetal toxicity, such as bone marrow suppression, ototoxicity, and gonadal depletion [15, 16]. Chemotherapy drugs that cross the placental barrier are metabolized mainly by the placenta. After the delivery, the newborn has a decreased capacity of drug metabolism. Hence, it is advisable to interrupt the chemotherapy from 2 to 3 weeks prior to the delivery, in order to prevent neonatal neutropenia or pancytopenia, neonatal sepsis, and bleeding disorders [3, 15, 16].

In turn, chronic leukemias have a less aggressive course and better perinatal outcomes. Women with chronic myeloid leukemia in major molecular response and reproductive desire should be counseled toward a planned conception after interrupting the intake of tyrosine kinase inhibitors (TKI).

Fetal exposure to imatinib in the first trimester is associated with a higher than expected incidence of skeletal, renal, respiratory, and gastrointestinal congenital abnormalities [4, 11, 17]. TKI should be discontinued before or at the moment of the diagnosis of pregnancy.

Women with chronic myeloid leukemias in the chronic phase frequently have uneventful pregnancies, achieving delivery at term [4, 11, 12, 17, 18]. However, chronic myeloid leukemia in accelerated phase or blastic phase has an aggressive course and poorer maternal-fetal outcomes, similar to those cases of acute leukemia.

Patients presenting with thrombocytosis (platelet count $> 500 \times 10^9$ /L) have an increased risk of thrombosis during pregnancy [4, 11]. Cases of hyperleukocytosis have been described among pregnant women with chronic leukemia after the TKI discontinuation [4, 11, 19].

5.3 Management of the Pregnancy Complicated by Leukemia

The management of pregnancies complicated by leukemia depends on the type of leukemia, gestational age, and on the balance of risks and benefits from chemotherapy versus expectant management. Pregnant women with leukemia should always be promptly referred to a specialized multidisciplinary team.

Cases of acute leukemia should be evaluated by the trimester of gestation. The first step is to perform an early endovaginal ultrasound assessment to accurately determine the gestational age.

5.3.1 First Trimester

The life expectancy of patients with untreated acute leukemia is shorter than the length of gestation [2, 10]; thus, it is not possible to postpone the treatment with chemotherapy. Besides, a successful pregnancy is unlikely after an untreated acute leukemia in the first trimester [2]. Fetal exposure to maternal chemotherapy during the organogenic period is known to be associated to miscarriage, fetal abnormalities, and stillbirth.

In such a situation, termination of pregnancy (TOP) should be discussed with the patient and her family [2, 11]. An elective TOP with cervical ripening medications followed by uterine aspiration seems to be a safer option to those patients, as it is performed in the inpatient setting with tight control of hemostasis and availability of blood transfusion.

5.3.2 Second and Early Third Trimesters

Patients who have been diagnosed with acute leukemia in the second trimester and in the early third trimester (<32–34 weeks of gestation) should be promptly referred to specific standard chemotherapy, accordingly to the current protocols for each type and subtype of leukemia (see Chap. 2) [4, 11, 18].

Pregnant women under chemotherapy should be followed by a high-risk prenatal care, with appointments every 2–3 weeks. It is important to assure adequate nutritional intake and oral supplementations with iron and folic acid. Patients under chemotherapy frequently receive high doses of corticosteroids, so they should be tightly screened for complications such as hypertensive syndromes and gestational diabetes.

Severe anemia in pregnancy increases the risks of preterm delivery, intrauterine growth restriction, stillbirth, neonatal death, and maternal mortality [20]. Cases complicated by severe anemia will need transfusional support with the aim of hemoglobin levels above 7.0 g/dL.

Antenatal care must also comprise a thorough assessment of fetal morphology, growth, and well-being. Evaluation of fetal morphology should include first trimester scan ($11–13^{+6}$ weeks), second trimester scan plus endovaginal assessment of cervical length (20–24 weeks), and fetal echocardiography (24–28 weeks).

It is fundamental to maintain a tight assessment of fetal growth and well-being. Although, there is no well-established protocol for fetal monitoring in patients under chemotherapy, it is reasonable to perform obstetric ultrasound to assess fetal growth every 2 weeks. Intrauterine growth restriction is defined as an estimated fetal weight below the tenth percentile for gestational age, and it is associated to an increased risk of placental insufficiency.

Fetal viability refers to a gestational age in which neonatal intensive care would be sufficient to the survival of an extreme prematurely delivered newborn. Clearly, this concept depends intrinsically on the available technological apparatus and staff expertise in each neonatal intensive care unit. Hence, every hospital has its own gestational age of fetal viability. Currently, the worldwide definition of fetal viability is around 24 to 26 weeks of gestation [21].

When the gestational age of fetal viability is reached, the antenatal care of pregnancies complicated by leukemia should also include tests of fetal well-being. It is advisable that fetal biophysical profile, nonstress test, and uterine artery Doppler assessment should be performed every 1 or 2 weeks after 24–26 weeks of gestation. Abnormalities of the fetal well-being must be carefully analyzed by maternal-fetal specialists, and severe cases might indicate patient hospitalization or even the anticipation of the delivery.

The planning of delivery must consider several factors, such as:

- Establishing a safe gestational age of birth
- Achieving adequate maternal levels of hemoglobin, neutrophils, and platelets
- Interrupting the chemotherapy 2 or 3 weeks prior to the delivery to prevent maternal and fetal bone marrow suppression at delivery
- Availability of transfusional support in cases of excessive bleeding
- Adequate maternal clinical status

In order to fulfill the abovementioned prerogatives, patients with acute leukemia are planned to be delivered at 32–34 weeks of gestation [2, 4, 11]. The management of cases presenting with spontaneous preterm labor or preterm premature rupture of membranes (PPROM) should be individualized. Considering the severity of the maternal disease, it is not advisable to attempt tocolysis in cases of preterm labor.

5.3.3 Third Trimester

This group comprises patients diagnosed with acute leukemia after 30–32 weeks of gestation. In such cases, it is reasonable to schedule the delivery at 32–34 weeks and start chemotherapy after the delivery, if the maternal clinical status is not compromised.

Delivery 2 weeks following chemotherapy may be coincident with the maternal-fetal bone marrow suppression period, which increases the risks of neonatal neutropenia or pancytopenia, neonatal sepsis, and bleeding disorders [3, 15, 16]. Hence, patients should never receive chemotherapy after 36 weeks of gestation, due to the impending risk of labor onset [2].

Patients with chronic leukemias are likely to have uneventful pregnancies [12, 19]. However, those patients should also be followed at a high-risk antenatal care. It is recommended to assess fetal growth monthly. The delivery is planned at 40 weeks of gestation.

5.4   Delivery Considerations

Pregnancies complicated by acute leukemia are likely to have a premature delivery. The main causes of prematurity in such a group are spontaneous preterm labor, abnormalities of fetal well-being, and a medical indication of the anticipation of delivery [12].

Preterm birth is defined as delivery prior to 37 weeks of gestation, and it is associated with neonatal morbidities and death [22, 23]. Premature newborns have an increased risk of respiratory distress syndrome, interventricular hemorrhage, necrotizing enterocolitis, retinopathy, cognitive impairment, and neonatal death [22, 23]. Regarding to neonatal outcomes, the earlier the preterm birth, the higher the odds of neonatal morbidity and mortality [22, 23].

Antenatal administration of corticosteroids for fetal lung maturation is widely known to have a major impact on the improvement of neonatal outcomes. It reduces the risk of respiratory distress syndrome by approximately 50% [24]. Besides, it also reduces the incidence of interventricular hemorrhage, necrotizing enterocolitis, and neonatal death [24].

The International Federation of Gynecology and Obstetrics (FIGO) recommends that antenatal corticosteroids should be considered for all pregnant women between 24 weeks and 34 weeks of gestation, who have an imminent risk of delivery [24]. Available regimens of antenatal corticosteroids for fetal lung maturation consist of [24]:

- Intramuscular Betamethasone: two doses of 12 mg, 24 hours apart **OR**
- Intramuscular dexamethasone: four doses of 6 mg, 12 hours apart

Every pregnant woman with acute leukemia should receive one course of antenatal corticosteroids prior to the scheduled delivery.

Recent studies have suggested that the administration of intravenous magnesium sulfate shortly before the preterm delivery might have a neuroprotective effect, preventing cerebral palsy [25, 26]. However, it is not a well-established practice worldwide.

Cases of preterm delivery before 32 weeks of gestation should be considered for magnesium sulfate according to institutional protocols.

In the general population, cesarean delivery is associated with higher maternal morbidity and mortality [27]. C-section is related to higher intrapartum bleeding and higher risk of puerperal complications, such as postpartum endometritis, pneumonia, longer hospital stays, and anemia [27].

In patients with leukemia, induction of labor and vaginal delivery is the preferred route of delivery [2, 28]. Elective C-section should be limited to cases with obstetric contraindications to vaginal delivery.

Regarding the delivery anesthesia, epidural analgesia is usually contraindicated in patients with severe neutropenia ($<1 \times 10^9/L$) or severe thrombocytopenia ($<80 \times 10^9/L$). In such cases, it is possible to perform intravenous opioid analgesia. If there is an indication of C-section, general anesthesia should be performed.

Pregnant women with leukemia will likely present with low levels of hemoglobin and platelets, so it is pivotal to adequately control the intra- and postpartum blood losses. An active management of the third period of labor by the administration of intramuscular or intravenous oxytocin soon after the baby is born is recommended [29].

Following delivery, a histological evaluation of the placenta should be performed. Although extremely rare, there are few descriptions of placental metastasis in pregnant women with leukemia [1, 13, 14].

The postpartum is the pregnancy period with the higher risk of VTE. Patients with leukemia must have a VTE risk assessment and be considered for a VTE prophylaxis strategy according to the platelet count. Options for VTE prevention include low-molecular-weight heparin and mechanical prophylaxis.

Breastfeeding is contraindicated in patients who will continue the chemotherapy after delivery. In regard to cases of chronic myeloid leukemia, the decision of breastfeeding depends on the indication of imatinib. If there is a hematological indication for reintroducing the TKI drugs, breastfeeding is contraindicated.

5.5   Contraception

Patients with chronic myeloid leukemia on TKIs should stop the medication before pregnancy. Besides, women with acute leukemia under chemotherapy must avoid pregnancy for 1–2 years after the treatment. Chemotherapy-based regimens currently used in leukemia treatment may have a deleterious impact on ovarian reserve and fertility. However, chemotherapy-induced amenorrhea can be just transient in some patients [30].

The postpartum period is an excellent opportunity to actively discuss contraceptive options with the patient. Patients may be markedly immunosuppressed during the leukemia treatment; thus, the use of condoms should be recommended to prevent sexually transmitted diseases (STD).

However, condoms' effectiveness depends on the couple skills. Couples who use condoms correctly in every act of sex will have a 2% rate of unintended pregnancy in the first year [31]. Conversely, couples who make the "typical use" of condoms have a 13% rate of pregnancies in the first year [31]. Patients should be warned about the use of condoms to prevent STDs, but they also need to associate themselves to another contraceptive method.

The choice of the contraceptive method must consider that patients under chemotherapy may have special particularities besides pregnancy prevention, such as increased risks of VTE, immunosuppression, and abnormal vaginal bleeding.

Currently, the most commonly available contraceptive methods are as follows:

- Combined oral contraceptives (COC)
- Progestin-only pills
- Progestin-only injectables
- Combined patch
- Combined vaginal ring
- Subdermal progestin implants
- Copper-bearing intrauterine device (IUD)
- Levonorgestrel intrauterine system (IUS)
- Sterilization

Combined contraceptives (oral, patch, and vaginal ring) consist of progestin and estrogen. The continuous use of combined contraceptives may have the beneficial effect of reducing or even stopping menstrual vaginal bleeding [30]. However, the administration of estrogen in cancer patients may increase the VTE risk. It is thus recommended to avoid the use of combined methods in patients with active cancer or who have been treated for cancer in the last 6 months [32, 33].

Progestin-only methods do not seem to increase the risk of VTE and may induce amenorrhea. Progestin intramuscular injectables must be avoided in patients with severe thrombocytopenia ($<50 \times 10^9$/L) [33]. Although safe and efficacious, subdermal implants may cause unpredictable vaginal bleeding in some patients and thus may not be the first option for patients with severe anemia and thrombocytopenia.

Intrauterine devices (copper and levonorgestrel) have a long duration of effectiveness. There is a concern about the risk of infection, following the intrauterine device insertion due to the immunosuppression, but there are actual data on the safety of the intrauterine devices in non-oncologic immunosuppressed patients (HIV/AIDS) [33]. One possible strategy to reduce the risk of infection during the insertion of the intrauterine device is to perform a screening to chlamydia and gonorrhea by PCR prior to the insertion of the device [32].

The advantages of levonorgestrel-IUS rely on its long-term effectiveness and the fact that it does not interact with another medications nor depends on the patient's adherence [33]. Furthermore, levonorgestrel-IUS reduces menstrual vaginal bleeding or even causes amenorrhea. On the other hand, copper IUDs may not be first option as they may increase the menstrual blood flow [33].

Sterilization may be an option for older patients who do not desire another pregnancy. It may be performed soon after the delivery. However, sterilization indication depends on local policies.

References

1. Albright CM, Wenstrom KD. Malignancies in pregnancy. Best Pract Res Clin Obstet Gynaecol. 2016;3:2–18.
2. Ali S, Jones GL, Culligan DJ, Marsden PJ, Russell N, Embleton ND, et al. British Committee for Standards in hematology. Guidelines for the diagnosis and management of acute myeloid leukaemia in pregnancy. Br J Hematol. 2015;170(4):487–95.
3. Salani R, Billingsley CC, Crafton SM. Cancer and pregnancy : an overview for obstetricians and gynecologists. Am J Obstet Gynecol. 2014;211(1):7–14.
4. Lishner M, Avivi I, Apperley JF, Evens AM, Fumagalli M, Nulman I, et al. Hematologic malignancies in pregnancy : management guidelines from an international consensus meeting. J Clin Oncol. 2016;34(5):501–8.
5. de Haas S, Ghossein-Doha C, van Kujik SM, van Drongelen J, Spaanderman ME. Physiological adaptation of maternal plasma volume during pregnancy: a systematic review and meta-analysis. Ultrasound Obstet Gynecol. 2017;49:177–87.
6. World Health Organization. WHO recommendations on antenatal care for a positive pregnancy experience, vol. 152. Geneva: WHO; 2016.
7. Kuvin S, Brecher G. Differential neutrophil counts in pregnancy. N Engl J Med. 1962;266:877–8.
8. Sivasankar R, Kumar RA, Baraz R, Collis RE. The white cell count in pregnancy and labour : a reference range. J Matern Fetal Neonatal Med. 2015;28(7):790–2.
9. Cines DB, Levine LD. Thrombocytopenia in pregnancy. Blood. 2018;130(21):2271–7.
10. Iseminger KA, Lewis MA. Ethical challenges in treating mother and fetus when cancer complicates. Obstet Gynecol Clin N Am. 1998;25(2):273–85.
11. Barzilai M, Avivi I, Amit O. Hematological malignancies during pregnancy. Mol Clin Oncol. 2019;10(1):3–9.
12. Nomura RM, Igai AM, Faciroli NC, Aguiar IN, Zugaib M. Maternal and perinatal outcomes in pregnant women with leukemia. Rev Bras Ginecol Obstet. 2011;33(8):174–81.
13. Osada S, Horibe K, Oiwa K, Yoshida J, Iwamura H, Matsuoka H, et al. A case of infantile acute monocytic leukemia caused by vertical transmission of the mother's leukemic cells. Cancer. 1990;65(5):1146–9.
14. Dessolle L, Dalmon C, Roche B, Daraï E. Placental metastases from maternal malignancies : review of the literature. J Gynecol Obstet Biol Reprod (Paris). 2007;36(4):344–53.
15. Ko EM, Van LeL. Chemotherapy for gynecologic cancers occurring during pregnancy. Obstet Gynecol Surv. 2011;66(5):291–8.
16. Brewer M, Kueck A, Runowicz CD. Chemotherapy in pregnancy. Clin Obstet Gynecol. 2011;54(4):602–18.
17. Dou X, Qin Y, Jiang Q. Planned pregnancy in female patients with chronic myeloid leukemia receiving tyrosine kinase inhibitor therapy. Oncologist. 2019;24(11):e1141–7.
18. Pallavee P, Samal R, Ghose S. Chronic myeloid leukaemia in pregnancy : call for guidelines. J Obstet Gynaecol. 2019;39(4):582–3.
19. Moura AC, Delamain MT, Duarte GBO, Lorand-Metze I. SouzaCA, Pagnano KBB. Management of chronic myeloid leukemia during pregnancy : a retrospective analysis at a single center. Hematol Transfus Cell Ther. 2019;41(2):125–8.
20. Jung J, Rahman MM, Rahman MS, Swe KT, Islam MR, Rahman MO, et al. Effects of hemoglobin levels during pregnancy on adverse maternal and infant outcomes : a systematic review and meta-analysis. Ann N Y Acad Sci. 2019;1450(1):69–82.
21. Breborowicz G. Limits of fetal viability and its enhancement. Early Pregnancy. 2001;5:49–50.
22. Frey HA, Klebanoff MA. The epidemiology, etiology, and costs of preterm birth. Semin Fetal Neonatal Med. 2016;21(2):68–73.
23. Harrison MS, Goldenberg RL. Global burden of prematurity. Semin Fetal Neonatal Med. 2015;21(2):74–9.

24. FIGO Working Group on Good Clinical Practice in Maternal-Fetal Medicine. Good clinical practice advice : antenatal corticosteroids for fetal lung maturation. Int J Gynaecol Obstet. 2019;144(3):352–5.
25. The American College of Obstetrics and Gynecologist Committee on Obstetric Practice Society for Maternal-Fetal Medicine. Committee opinion No 652: magnesium sulfate use in obstetrics. Obstet Gynecol. 2016;127(1):e52-3: 12–3.
26. Royal College of Obstetricians and Gynaecologists. Magnesium sulphate to prevent cerebral palsy following preterm birth. Scientific Impact Paper No. 29 2011.
27. Buhimschi CS, Buhimschi IA. Advantages of vaginal delivery. Clin Obstet Gynaecol. 2006;49(1):167–83.
28. Rizack T, Mega A, Legare R, Castillo J. Management of hematological malignancies during pregnancy. Am J Hematol. 2009;84(12):830–41.
29. World Health Organization. Active management of the third stage of labor. New WHO recommendations help to focus implementation.New WI. Active management of the third new WHO recommendations help to focus implementation. Geneva: WHO; 2013.
30. Cagnacci A, Ramirez I, Bitzer J, Gompel A. Contraception in cancer survivors – an expert review part II. Skin, gastrointestinal, haematological and endocrine cancers. Eur J Contracept Reprod Health Care. 2019;24(4):299–304.
31. World Health Organization Department of Reproductive Health and Research (WHO / RHR) and Johns Hopkins Bloomberg School of Public Health / Center for Communication Programs (CCP), Knowledge for Health Project. Family planning: a global handbook for providers (2018 update). Baltimore/Geneva: CCP and WHO; 2018.
32. Pragout D, Laurence V, Baffet H, Raccah-Tebeka B, Rousset-Jablonski C. Contraception and cancer : CNGOF contraception guidelines. Gynecol Obstet Fertil Senol. 2018;46(12):834–44.
33. Society of Family Planning. Cancer and contraception. Contraception. 2012;86:191–8.

Chapter 6
Antibiotic and Antifungal Therapies During Leukemia Treatment in Pregnancy

Bruno Azevedo Randi and Vinicius Ponzio da Silva

6.1 Introduction

Drug prescription during pregnancy requires a delicate assessment of the balance between maternal benefit and fetal risks, including fetal loss, congenital malformations, organ toxicity, and prematurity [1]. The major infection complication during leukemia treatment is febrile neutropenia. In a small cohort of pregnant women with acute leukemia, 57.1% of them developed at least one episode of febrile neutropenia [2].

6.2 Febrile Neutropenia

One of the most frequent infection complications of chemotherapy is febrile neutropenia. Febrile neutropenia is defined as an oral temperature of > 38.3 °C or two consecutives readings of > 38.0 °C for 2 hours and an absolute neutrophil count of $< 0.5 \times 10^9$/L or expected to fall below 0.5×10^9/L within the following 48 hours. It is a major cause of mortality and morbidity, prolonging hospital stay, and increasing health costs [3]. The mortality levels can reach up to 50% [4]. Furthermore, it can delay the oncology treatment and impact the oncological outcome of the patient.

Prognosis is worse in cases of proven bacteremia. Bacteremia can be detected in 20% of cases of febrile neutropenia. Mortality rates vary from 18% in Gram-negative to 5% in Gram-positive bacteremia [5].

Individuals with febrile neutropenia can be classified as low-risk, intermediate-risk, and high-risk neutropenic patients based on underlying disease and type of treatment. The Multinational Association for Supportive Care of Cancer (MASCC)

B. A. Randi (✉) · V. P. da Silva
Hospital 9 de Julho, São Paulo, Brazil

© Springer Nature Switzerland AG 2021
C. W. P. Schmidt, K. M. Otoni (eds.), *Chemotherapy and Pharmacology for Leukemia in Pregnancy*, https://doi.org/10.1007/978-3-030-54058-6_6

risk index can be used to assess the necessity of hospitalization, which allocates points according to the importance of each variable: asymptomatic patient; patient presenting mild, moderate, or severe symptoms; no hypotension; no chronic obstructive pulmonary disease; solid tumor with no previous fungal infection; no dehydration; outpatient status at onset of fever; and age under 60 years. The MASCC risk index has a maximum score of 26 points and classifies the patients into low risk (≥21 points) or high risk (<21 points). It is widely used and considered to be simple, while presenting good sensitivity and a high positive value [4, 5]. Patients considered to be high risk should receive broad-spectrum intravenous antibiotic therapy (ABT) and indicated for hospitalization; patients with low risk and intermediate risk of complications may be considered candidates for ABT orally or intravenously and without hospitalization [4, 5].

6.3 Antibacterial Prophylaxis

Antibiotics have been used for a long time for the prevention of febrile neutropenia in patients under chemotherapy. This was a successful strategy but led to the emergence of resistant strains, limiting its efficacy. Guidelines from the European Organisation for Research and Treatment of Cancer (EORTC) and American Society of Clinical Oncology (ASCO) recommend that clinicians limit the use of antibacterial prophylaxis to patients at high risk for febrile neutropenia [5, 6].

6.4 Management of Febrile Neutropenia

A prompt recognition and reaction to a potential infection in the management of febrile neutropenia is required. The evaluation of the patient includes the following:

- Complete anamnesis with epidemiological investigation. Evaluate clinical records for past positive microbiology results (colonization and infections), vaccination, type of chemotherapy, antimicrobials used, and previous episodes of febrile neutropenia.
- Check the presence of catheters.
- Symptoms and signs that could suggest an infection focus (in the respiratory system, gastrointestinal tract, skin, perineal region, oropharynx, and central nervous system).
- Full physical exam, including oral cavity, skin, nails, and genital region. Avoid rectal touch.

Tests in the routine investigation include blood count, renal and liver function, coagulation screen, C-reactive protein, blood cultures (minimum of two sets, including from catheters), urinalysis and urine culture, and chest radiography. A skin biopsy should be considered if the patient has new skin lesions. With profound or prolonged neutropenia occurs, high-resolution computed topographies should be considered, and empirical antifungal therapy may be needed [5, 6].

6.5 Choice of IV Antibiotics

Local epidemiology bacterial resistance is essential in determining the first-choice empirical therapy. An increase in antibiotic-resistant strains has been reported, such as extended-spectrum beta-lactamase (ESBL) Gram-negative bacteria, carbapenem-resistant enterobacteria, vancomycin-resistant enterococci (VRE), and methicillin-resistant *Staphylococcus aureus* (MRSA) [5, 6].

Therefore, it is impossible to assemble one single guideline for everyone to use. When treating a pregnant woman with febrile neutropenia during the leukemia treatment, the physician should take into account:

- The local epidemiology
- The MASSC risk score
- The pregnancy category of antibiotics and antifungal drugs planned to be use
- Previous colonization, antibiotic used, and febrile neutropenia episodes
- Site of infection
- Comorbidities
- Severity and organ failure

Figure 6.1 presents a suggestion for antibiotic empirical treatment in pregnant women with febrile neutropenia during leukemia treatment.

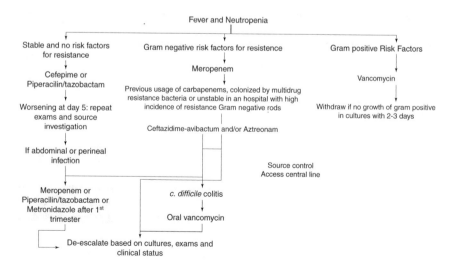

Fig. 6.1 Suggestion for antibiotic empirical treatment in pregnant women with febrile neutropenia during leukemia treatment

6.6 Pregnancy Category

The US Food and Drug Administration (FDA) previously categorized pregnancy risk in five categories [3, 7]:

- A: No risk in human studies. Adequate and well-controlled human studies have failed to demonstrate a risk to the fetus in the first trimester of pregnancy (and there is no evidence of risk in later trimesters).
- B: No risk in other studies. Animal reproduction studies have failed to demonstrate a risk to the fetus, and there are no adequate and well-controlled studies in pregnant women.
- C: Risk not ruled out. Animal reproduction studies have shown an adverse effect on the fetus, and there are no adequate and well-controlled studies in humans, but potential benefits may warrant use of the drug in pregnant women despite potential risks.
- D: Positive evidence of risk. There is positive evidence of human fetal risk, based on adverse reaction data from investigational or marketing experience or studies in humans, but potential benefits may warrant use of the drug in pregnant women despite potential risks.
- X: Contraindicated in pregnancy. Studies in animals or humans have demonstrated fetal abnormalities, and/or there is positive evidence of human fetal risk, based on adverse reaction data from investigational or marketing experience, and the risks involved in use of the drug in pregnant women clearly outweigh potential benefits

The FDA amended its rules in 2015 concerning the "Pregnancy," "Labor and delivery," and "Nursing mothers" subsections of the "Use in specific populations" section of product labeling. Pregnancy categories A, B, C, D, and X have been removed. Drugs approved after June 30 will use the new format immediately, while drugs approved after June 30, 2011, will be phased in gradually [7].

6.7 Antibiotics

Although use of any medication during pregnancy is a risk-versus-benefit decision, untreated infections are associated with significant fetal risk, including spontaneous abortion, prematurity, and low birth weight [8, 9]. Besides that, as was already discussed, febrile neutropenia is a medical emergency with high mortality and morbidity. Many antibiotics are considered safe in pregnancy, especially beta-lactams, macrolides, clindamycin, and fosfomycin; however, additional data are needed for the majority of antibiotic classes [3].

6.8 Beta-Lactams

6.8.1 Penicillins

Penicillins cross the placenta in high concentration. Due to increased plasma volume and creatinine clearance in pregnant women, serum penicillin concentrations may be decreased by as much as 50% [10]. Penicillins have strong evidence of safety during pregnancy, with the natural penicillin and the aminopenicillins (ampicillin and amoxicillin) having the most robust data [9]. All penicillins, their derivates, and the association with beta-lactamase inhibitors (e.g., clavulanate and sulbactam) have been classified as Pregnancy Category B [3].

6.8.2 Cephalosporins

The antibiotics of the class of cephalosporins have a long history of documented use in pregnancy [11]. Cephalosporins have decreased plasma concentrations in pregnant women due to increased renal elimination [3]. All cephalosporins are classified as Pregnancy Category B [3], including newly approved agents such as ceftaroline, ceftolozone-tazobactam, and ceftazidime-avibactam. Some studies suggest a potential association between ceftriaxone and cardiac malformation [3].

6.8.3 Carbapenems

There is a lack of data of the use of carbapenems in pregnant women. While ertapenem, meropenem, and doripenem are classified as Pregnancy Category Risk B, imipenem is Pregnancy Category C [3].

6.8.4 Monobactams

Aztreonam has inconclusive data regarding the safety of its use during pregnancy. Most studies are from the perinatal period; thus, this antibiotic should be used with caution during the first trimester as data are limited [3].

6.9   Aminoglycosides

The main aminoglycosides are amikacin, gentamicin, streptomycin, and tobramycin. During pregnancy, the serum half-life of this antibiotics is shorter, with an increase in the antibiotic's clearance. Moreover, pregnancy leads to a large volume of distribution, and this can lead to a lower serum peak concentration compared to nonpregnant women [3].

They can cross the human placenta and may result in fetus toxicities, especially when they are administered in the first trimester of pregnancy [3]. Some case reports of irreversible bilateral congenital deafness after maternal use of streptomycin in the first trimester lead to a boxed warning and an FDA Pregnancy Category of D for the class [3, 11]. A similar hearing loss has not been commonly associated with other aminoglycosides: if hearing abnormalities did occur, symptoms were mild or without clinical significance [3, 9, 12].

6.10   Fluoroquinolones

Although these antibiotics are classified as Pregnancy Category C, they are generally contraindicated in pregnancy [3]. They are widely distributed in the body, and protein binding can range from 20% to 50% [3]. Quinolones may be safe in the first trimester, but they are not recommended because they were associated with fetal harm in previous animal studies [8, 9, 13]. Some data link the use of fluoroquinolones in pregnancy with renal toxicity, cardiac defects, and central nervous system toxicity in rats [14, 15], but more studies are needed to confirm these associations. Animal data also showed bone and cartilage damage in fetus [3].

6.11   Glycopeptides and Lipoglycopeptides

Vancomycin is a glycopeptide thought to be safe for use in pregnancy in the case of serious Gram-positive infections [3]. This antibiotic is classified as Pregnancy Category B. Vancomycin is widely distributed in body tissues and eliminated by glomerular filtration in kidneys [3]. There are case reports that suggest the safety of vancomycin in pregnant women [12, 16]. In animal trials, no congenital malformations were noted after intravenous administration of vancomycin in rats and rabbits [3].

The lipoglycopeptides are represented by telavancin, oritavancin, and dalbavancin. They have similar Gram-positive activity when compared to vancomycin [3]. Animal data suggest that telavancin can be toxic, and, thus, it is classified as Pregnancy Risk C [3]. Telavancin caused limb and skeletal malformations and fetal weight loss in rat and rabbit studies. There is lack of human data [3]. Oritavancin showed no fetus toxicity in rat and rabbit studies. Dalbavancin exposure in rats showed no increase in embryo lethality [3].

6.12 Macrolides

Data regarding the use of macrolides in pregnant women are variable [3]. Macrolides have low protein binding, large volume of distribution, and hepatic metabolism. Thus, the physiologic changes of pregnancy have less impact on the kinetics of macrolides [3]. These drugs are represented by erythromycin, azithromycin, and clarithromycin.

In a retrospective study with 1033 pregnant women that used macrolides, there was no association with major malformations in the fetus. Also, exposure in the third trimester was not associated with pyloric stenosis or intussusception [3].

In another study that reviewed maternal erythromycin exposure of over 15 years, erythromycin was associated with cardiovascular defects. Despite that, most of the defects were mild [17].

Azithromycin usually is considered safe to use in pregnancy and is classified as Pregnancy Category B. In rats and mice, azithromycin was not associated with fetal harm [18].

Clarithromycin is classified as Pregnancy Category C. In animal studies, some rats exposed to this antibiotic in the first trimester did not result in malformations, while other rats showed low incidences of cardiac abnormalities after clarithromycin exposure [18]. Other studies also report cleft palate in murine models and retarded fetal growth in monkeys [18]. But in clinical data, including one prospective controlled study, clarithromycin was not linked to major malformations [10, 19, 20]. Despite the conflicting data, it is thought that azithromycin is safe to use during pregnancy, and clarithromycin should be used with caution and only when benefit outweighs risk [3].

6.13 Oxazolidinones

There is a lack of pharmacokinetic and controlled studies of linezolid and tedizolid in pregnant women. A case report showed positive maternal outcomes without fetus teratogenesis with 4 weeks of linezolid use starting at 14 weeks of pregnancy [14]. Studies on mice, rats, and rabbits have not shown teratogenic effects [3]. In rats, linezolid and tedizolid resulted in mild fetal toxicities, including decreased fetal body weight and reduced ossification on the sternebra [3]. Both linezolid and tedizolid are Pregnancy Category C.

6.14   Tetracyclines

Tetracyclines (minocycline, doxycycline, and tetracycline) are classified as Pregnancy Category D because of proven teratogenicity in humans [3]. They are associated with congenital defects and high doses with maternal liver toxicity [3]. Tetracyclines cross the placenta and when used beyond the second trimester can bind to calcium in the fetus. This can cause permanent discoloration of bones and teeth [3].

6.15   Daptomycin

Daptomycin is a cyclic lipopeptide used for treatment of Gram-positive infections. There are no controlled trials with this antibiotic in pregnancy, but some reports (one *Enterococcus faecium* pyelonephritis and one tricuspid valve endocarditis) suggest that its use can be safe [21, 22]. No patient or neonate adverse events are noted in both of the records. Administration of daptomycin in rats and rabbits showed no evidence of harm to fetus.

6.16   Fidaxomicin

Fidaxomicin is a macrocyclic, nonabsorbable antibiotic. It is classified as Pregnancy Category B, but there are no published studies about its use in pregnant women [3]. Studies in rabbits and rats showed no harm to fetus. Most patients have undetectable levels of fidaxomicin in plasma [23].

6.17   Metronidazole

Although metronidazole is classified as Pregnancy Category B, it cannot be used in the first trimester of pregnancy [3]. A lot of trials have linked metronidazole use with increased preterm birth rates [24, 25]. Vaginal metronidazole should be used with caution in pregnant women because some data suggested a link between its use and congenital hydrocephalus [26].

6.18   Clindamycin

This antibiotic belongs to the lincosamide family. It can cross the placenta and is classified as Pregnancy Category B. Clindamycin is distributed in most tissues and has high plasma protein bound [3]. In a study comprising 647 newborns who had been exposed to clindamycin during the first trimester of pregnancy did not support an association between congenital defects and the use of the drug [3].

6.19 Fosfomycin

Fosfomycin is classified as Pregnancy Category B. It is a well-tolerated antibiotic. Fosfomycin can cross the placenta barrier, but no adverse events in fetus or infant have been reported [27]. In Europe, it is used with caution as an injectable antimicrobial, which is not available either in United States or in Brazil [27]. Oral fosfomycin can be used in the treatment of lower urinary tract infections due to its high sensitivity on most bacteria (including multidrug-resistant organisms) and safety in pregnancy [3].

6.20 Nitrofurantoin

Nitrofurantoin, an antibiotic for urinary tract infections, is classified as Pregnancy Category B [3]. In animal studies, exposure to nitrofurantoin did not result in teratogenic effects. In a meta-analysis, no major malformation was associated with nitrofurantoin use in pregnant women [28]. It is important to remember that the use of this antibiotic may increase the risk of hemolytic anemia in pregnant patients with severe glucose-6-phosphate dehydrogenase deficiency [3].

6.21 Tigecycline

Tigecycline is classified as a glycylcycline. It can cross the placenta barrier and is classified as Pregnancy Category D [3]. Animal data showed several adverse outcomes, like fetal loss and possible discoloration of infant's teeth. There are no human studies to date [3].

6.22 Polymyxins

Polymyxin B and polymyxin E (colistin) are classified as Pregnancy Category C [3]. In animal models, polymyxin B showed toxic effects to the embryo [29]. There are few published cases of polymyxin use in pregnant women. In these studies, there is no evidence in the increase of preterm birth, low birth weight, and congenital abnormalities [3]. Thus, the lack of data on polymyxins' use in pregnant women and the high potential for adverse effects may lead to strong caution prior to use [3].

6.23   Sulfamethoxazole-Trimethoprim

Both sulfamethoxazole and trimethoprim are classified as Pregnant Category C [3]. Animal models observed teratogenic effects. Both the antibiotics cross the placenta barrier and should be avoided mainly in the first trimester because of the effect of trimethoprim as a folate antagonist: this could significantly raise the risk of neural tube and cardiac defects [30]. Increase in cardiac and limb malformations were observed with trimethoprim use 12 weeks prior to conception [31]. Besides that, the maternal supplementation of folic acid reduces major malformations induced by trimethoprim [3].

Sulfonamides theoretically result in unbound bilirubin in the third trimester due to competitive protein binding [3]. Also, the use of sulfamethoxazole-trimethoprim in the first trimester has been associated with an increase of urinary tract defects, and its use during the last two trimesters has been small for gestational age newborns [30, 32].

6.24   Antimycobacterial Agents

The first-line therapy for tuberculosis in pregnant women is the same for general population, including isoniazid, rifampin, ethambutol, and pyrazinamide [3, 33]. There is a systematic review showing safety of the first-line therapy in pregnant women [33]. Rifampin in animal studies did not show fetal abnormalities. This was also observed in more than 2000 pregnant women [34]. Ethambutol is associated with retrobulbar neuritis in the general population but has not been associated to either pregnant women or infants born from mothers exposed to ethambutol during pregnancy [34]. There are no reports of controlled studies to validate the safety of pyrazinamide during pregnancy, but case reports showed no fetal harm [3]. The antituberculosis agent, bedaquiline, is considered as a Pregnancy Category B [3].

Table 6.1 indicates the pregnancy category for each antibiotic.

6.25   Antifungals

Because pregnancy is a duly established contraindication for controlled studies, involving antifungal drugs, data in this setting are limited and based on in vitro or animal studies, pharmacological investigations, case reports, and expert opinions [1].

Table 6.1 Main antibiotics and its pregnancy category, as classified by the US Food and Drug Administration (FDA) [3, 7]

Drug	Pregnancy category
Amikacin	D
Amoxicillin-Clavulanate	B
Aztreonam	B
Azithromycin	B
Cefepime	B
Ceftazidime	B
Ceftazidime-Avibactam	B
Cefuroxime	B
Ciprofloxacin	C
Clarithromycin	C
Clindamycin	B
Daptomycin	B
Fidaxomicin	B
Fosfomycin	B
Gentamicin	D
Imipenem	C
Levofloxacin	C
Linezolid	C
Meropenem	B
Metronidazole	B
Nitrofurantoin	B
Piperacillin-tazobactam	B
Polymyxin B	C
Polymyxin E (Colistin)	C
Trimethoprim-sulfamethoxazole	C
Tedizolid	C
Teicoplanin	B
Tigecycline	Humans: may cause fetal harm Animals: fetal toxicity
Vancomycin	C

6.26 Systemic Azoles

Azoles include imidazoles and triazoles. The mechanism of action targets the C14 alpha demethylase and thereby inhibits the biosynthesis of ergosterol, an essential component of fungal cell membranes. Animal and human data show that azoles could be teratogenic [1].

Fluconazole is a systemic triazole with fungistatic effect on yeasts like *Candida* sp. and *Cryptococcus* sp. It can cross the placenta and was shown to be embryotoxic in rabbits and teratogenic in rats [1, 35]. Some reports of congenital abnormalities in children exposed during pregnancy have been reported [1, 36–38] with the dose of 400 mg/day or above during the first trimester. Lesions described include trapezoidocephaly, midfacial hypoplasia, cartilage abnormalities with multiple synostoses, and skeletal fractures [1].

Itraconazole is a triazole with spectrum of activity that includes endemic fungi and *Aspergillus* species. It is embryotoxic and teratogenic in rodents, including craniofacial and rib abnormalities [1]. A higher rate of early fetal loss was reported (12% versus 4% in the control group) [1, 39].

Voriconazole is a triazole with fungistatic activity against *Candida* sp. and fungicidal activity against *Aspergillus fumigatus*. Voriconazole is teratogenic in rodents with high and also lower doses. Visceral and skeletal abnormalities were reported [1]. There are data of embryo/fetotoxicity in rabbits. Since its approval by the FDA in 2002, only one report of voriconazole exposure in pregnancy has been reported, with good maternal-fetal outcome [1, 40].

Posaconazole is a triazole with expanded antifungal spectrum, including *Mucorales*. Teratogenic effects have been reported in rats (skeletal malformations and rib abnormalities). It was also shown to be embryotoxic and teratogenic in rabbits [1].

Isavuconazole is the newest azole with broad spectrum. To date, no human data are available regarding its use during pregnancy [1].

6.27 Equinocandins

The antifungals of this class act by inhibiting the 1,3-beta-D-glucan synthesis, involved in fungal wall synthesis. The antifungals of this class are caspofungin, micafungin, and anidulafungin. They have broad spectrum of action, which includes *Candida* spp. and *Aspergillus* spp. They cross the placenta of rats and rabbits, being embryotoxic and teratogenic [1]. Besides that, they can cross the human placenta [1]. Both caspofungin and micafungin are classified as Pregnant Category C, whereas anidulafungin is Category B [3].

6.28 Flucytosine

Flucytosine is converted in fungal cells in fluorouracil, interfering with both DNA and protein synthesis. The spectrum is limited to yeasts, including *Candida* spp. and *Cryptococcus* spp. Flucytosine is teratogenic in rats and crosses the human placenta, achieving high concentration in amniotic fluid and cord blood. It is embryotoxic and teratogenic in rodents, but not in monkeys [1]. Fetuses exposed in the first trimester can develop structural abnormalities [1]. Seven cases reports have been published, describing good maternal-fetal outcomes, following administration during pregnancy [41–43]. They come under Pregnancy Category is C [3].

6.29 Systemic Polyenes

Polyenes binds to ergosterol, forming transmembrane pores, leading to ionic leakage and fungal death. Amphotericin B has a large fungal spectrum, which includes yeasts and mounds, including *Mucorales* and dimorphic fungi. Amphotericin B is the systemic antifungal drug treatment, which has been used extensively during pregnancy, with no reports of teratogenesis attributed to it and Pregnancy Category is B [3]. Maternal nephrotoxicity is similar to that in nonpregnant patients [1, 41].

Thus, Amphotericin B and its lipidic formulations are the cornerstones of treatment of any invasive fungal infection during pregnancy [1]. Table 6.2 indicates the pregnancy category for each antifungal. Table 6.3 shows the indicative treatment for each invasive fungal disease in pregnant women.

Table 6.2 Main antifungals and their pregnancy categories, as classified by the US Food and Drug Administration (FDA) [7]

Drug	Pregnancy category
Amphotericin B	B
Fluconazole	C (single dose) D (other regimens)
Itraconazole	C
Voriconazole	D
Posaconazole	C
Isavuconazole	C
Anidulafungin	B
Caspofungin	C
Micafungin	C

Table 6.3 Main fungal disease treatments during pregnancy, based on practice guidelines

Disease	Term of pregnancy		Alternative proposition
	First trimester	Second–third trimester	
Coccidioidomycosis	Amphotericin B lipid formulation 2–5 mg/kg/day or Amphotericin B deoxycholate 0.5–1.5 mg/kg/day	Amphotericin B lipid formulation 2–5 mg/kg/day	–
Aspergillosis	No specific recommendation on practice guidelines	No specific recommendation on practice guidelines	–
Disseminated cryptococcosis	Amphotericin B lipid formulation 2–5 mg/kg/day or Amphotericin B deoxycholate 0.5–1.5 mg/kg/day ± flucytosine	Amphotericin B lipid formulation 2–5 mg/kg/day or Amphotericin B deoxycholate 0.5–1.5 mg/kg/day ± flucytosine	Fluconazole should ideally be started after delivery, and, if not possible, after the first trimester

(continued)

Table 6.3 (conitnued)

Disease	Term of pregnancy		Alternative proposition
	First trimester	Second–third trimester	
Blastomycosis	Amphotericin B lipid formulation 2-5 mg/kg/day	Amphotericin B lipid formulation 2-5 mg/kg/day	
Histoplasmosis	Amphotericin B lipid formulation 2–5 mg/kg/day	Amphotericin B lipid formulation 2–5 mg/kg/day	Amphotericin B deoxycholate 0.5–1.5 mg/kg/day
Invasive candidiasis	Amphotericin B lipid formulation 2–5 mg/kg/day or Amphotericin B deoxycholate 0.5–1.5 mg/kg/day	Amphotericin B lipid formulation 2–5 mg/kg/day or Amphotericin B deoxycholate 0.5–1.5 mg/kg/day	
Sporotrichosis	Amphotericin B lipid formulation 2–5 mg/kg/day or Amphotericin B deoxycholate 0.7–1 mg/kg/day	Amphotericin B lipid formulation 2–5 mg/kg/day or Amphotericin B deoxycholate 0.7–1 mg/kg/day	

Adapted from Pilmis et al. [1, 44–51]

References

1. Pilmis B, Jullien V, Sobel J, Lecuit M, Lortholary O, Charlier C. Antifungal drugs during pregnancy: an updated review. J Antimicrob Chemother. 2015;70(1):14–22.
2. Nomura RMY. Resultados maternos e perinatais em gestantes portadoras de leucemia. Rev Bras Ginecol. 2011;33:174–81.
3. Bookstaver PB, Bland CM, Griffin B, Stover KR, Eiland LS, McLaughlin M. A review of antibiotic use in pregnancy. Pharmacotherapy. 2015;35(11):1052–62.
4. Ferreira JN. Managing febrile neutropenia in adult cancer patients: an integrative review of the literature. Rev Bras Enferm. 2017;70:1301–8.
5. Klastersky J, de Naurois J, Rolston K, Rapoport B, Maschmeyer G, Aapro M, et al. Management of febrile neutropaenia: ESMO clinical practice guidelines. Ann Oncol. 2016;27(suppl 5):v111–v8.
6. Taplitz RA, Kennedy EB, Flowers CR. Outpatient management of fever and neutropenia in adults treated for malignancy: American Society of Clinical Oncology and Infectious Diseases Society of America clinical practice guideline update summary. J Oncol Pract. 2018;14(4):250–5.
7. Gilbert DN. The Sanford guide to antimicrobial therapy 2019. Sperryville: Antimicrobial Therapy, Inc; 2019.
8. Harbison AF, Polly DM, Musselman ME. Antiinfective therapy for pregnant or lactating patients in the emergency department. Am J Health Syst Pharm. 2015;72(3):189–97.
9. Lamont HF, Blogg HJ, Lamont RF. Safety of antimicrobial treatment during pregnancy: a current review of resistance, immunomodulation and teratogenicity. Expert Opin Drug Saf. 2014;13(12):1569–81.
10. Einarson A, Shuhaiber S, Koren G. Effects of antibacterials on the unborn child: what is known and how should this influence prescribing. Paediatr Drugs. 2001;3(11):803–16.

11. Heikkilä AM. Antibiotics in pregnancy--a prospective cohort study on the policy of antibiotic prescription. Ann Med. 1993;25(5):467–71.
12. Adam MP, Polifka JE, Friedman JM. Evolving knowledge of the teratogenicity of medications in human pregnancy. Am J Med Genet C Semin Med Genet. 2011;157C(3):175–82.
13. Yefet E, Salim R, Chazan B, Akel H, Romano S, Nachum Z. The safety of quinolones in pregnancy. Obstet Gynecol Surv. 2014;69(11):681–94.
14. Guinto VT, De Guia B, Festin MR, Dowswell T. Different antibiotic regimens for treating asymptomatic bacteriuria in pregnancy. Cochrane Database Syst Rev. 2010;(9):CD007855.
15. Crider KS, Cleves MA, Reefhuis J, Berry RJ, Hobbs CA, Hu DJ. Antibacterial medication use during pregnancy and risk of birth defects: National Birth Defects Prevention Study. Arch Pediatr Adolesc Med. 2009;163(11):978–85.
16. Reyes MP, Ostrea EM, Cabinian AE, Schmitt C, Rintelmann W. Vancomycin during pregnancy: does it cause hearing loss or nephrotoxicity in the infant? Am J Obstet Gynecol. 1989;161(4):977–81.
17. Källén B, Danielsson BR. Fetal safety of erythromycin. An update of Swedish data. Eur J Clin Pharmacol. 2014;70(3):355–60.
18. Amsden GW. Erythromycin, clarithromycin, and azithromycin: are the differences real? Clin Ther. 1996;18(1):56–72; discussion 55.
19. Drinkard CR, Shatin D, Clouse J. Postmarketing surveillance of medications and pregnancy outcomes: clarithromycin and birth malformations. Pharmacoepidemiol Drug Saf. 2000;9(7):549–56.
20. Einarson A, Phillips E, Mawji F, D'Alimonte D, Schick B, Addis A, et al. A prospective controlled multicentre study of clarithromycin in pregnancy. Am J Perinatol. 1998;15(9):523–5.
21. Shea K, Hilburger E, Baroco A, Oldfield E. Successful treatment of vancomycin-resistant Enterococcus faecium pyelonephritis with daptomycin during pregnancy. Ann Pharmacother. 2008;42(5):722–5.
22. Stroup JS, Wagner J, Badzinski T. Use of daptomycin in a pregnant patient with Staphylococcus aureus endocarditis. Ann Pharmacother. 2010;44(4):746–9.
23. Sears P, Crook DW, Louie TJ, Miller MA, Weiss K. Fidaxomicin attains high fecal concentrations with minimal plasma concentrations following oral administration in patients with Clostridium difficile infection. Clin Infect Dis. 2012;55(Suppl 2):S116–20.
24. Ramsey PS, Andrews WW. Biochemical predictors of preterm labor: fetal fibronectin and salivary estriol. Clin Perinatol. 2003;30(4):701–33.
25. Klebanoff MA, Carey JC, Hauth JC, Hillier SL, Nugent RP, Thom EA, et al. Failure of metronidazole to prevent preterm delivery among pregnant women with asymptomatic Trichomonas vaginalis infection. N Engl J Med. 2001;345(7):487–93.
26. Kazy Z, Puhó E, Czeizel AE. Teratogenic potential of vaginal metronidazole treatment during pregnancy. Eur J Obstet Gynecol Reprod Biol. 2005;123(2):174–8.
27. Keating GM. Fosfomycin trometamol: a review of its use as a single-dose oral treatment for patients with acute lower urinary tract infections and pregnant women with asymptomatic bacteriuria. Drugs. 2013;73(17):1951–66.
28. Goldberg O, Moretti M, Levy A, Koren G. Exposure to nitrofurantoin during early pregnancy and congenital malformations: a systematic review and meta-analysis. J Obstet Gynaecol Can. 2015;37(2):150–6.
29. Jaiswal MK, Agrawal V, Jaiswal YK. Effect of polymyxin B on gram-negative bacterial infection during pregnancy. J Turk Ger Gynecol Assoc. 2011;12(2):64–70.
30. Matok I, Gorodischer R, Koren G, Landau D, Wiznitzer A, Levy A. Exposure to folic acid antagonists during the first trimester of pregnancy and the risk of major malformations. Br J Clin Pharmacol. 2009;68(6):956–62.
31. Andersen JT, Petersen M, Jimenez-Solem E, Rasmussen JN, Andersen NL, Afzal S, et al. Trimethoprim use prior to pregnancy and the risk of congenital malformation: a register-based nationwide cohort study. Obstet Gynecol Int. 2013;2013:364526.

32. Santos F, Sheehy O, Perreault S, Ferreira E, Berard A. Exposure to anti-infective drugs during pregnancy and the risk of small-for-gestational-age newborns: a case-control study. BJOG. 2011;118(11):1374–82.
33. Nguyen HT, Pandolfini C, Chiodini P, Bonati M. Tuberculosis care for pregnant women: a systematic review. BMC Infect Dis. 2014;14:617.
34. Bothamley G. Drug treatment for tuberculosis during pregnancy: safety considerations. Drug Saf. 2001;24(7):553–65.
35. Tiboni GM. Second branchial arch anomalies induced by fluconazole, a bis-triazole antifungal agent, in cultured mouse embryos. Res Commun Chem Pathol Pharmacol. 1993;79(3):381–4.
36. Aleck KA, Bartley DL. Multiple malformation syndrome following fluconazole use in pregnancy: report of an additional patient. Am J Med Genet. 1997;72(3):253–6.
37. Pursley TJ, Blomquist IK, Abraham J, Andersen HF, Bartley JA. Fluconazole-induced congenital anomalies in three infants. Clin Infect Dis. 1996;22(2):336–40.
38. Lee BE, Feinberg M, Abraham JJ, Murthy AR. Congenital malformations in an infant born to a woman treated with fluconazole. Pediatr Infect Dis J. 1992;11(12):1062–4.
39. Bar-Oz B, Moretti ME, Bishai R, Mareels G, Van Tittelboom T, Verspeelt J, et al. Pregnancy outcome after in utero exposure to itraconazole: a prospective cohort study. Am J Obstet Gynecol. 2000;183(3):617–20.
40. Bitar D, Morizot G, Van Cauteren D, Dannaoui E, Lanternier F, Lortholary O, et al. Estimating the burden of mucormycosis infections in France (2005–2007) through a capture-recapture method on laboratory and administrative data. Rev Epidemiol Sante Publique. 2012;60(5):383–7.
41. Moudgal VV, Sobel JD. Antifungal drugs in pregnancy: a review. Expert Opin Drug Saf. 2003;2(5):475–83.
42. Ely EW, Peacock JE, Haponik EF, Washburn RG. Cryptococcal pneumonia complicating pregnancy. Medicine (Baltimore). 1998;77(3):153–67.
43. Costa ML, Souza JP, Oliveira Neto AF, Pinto E Silva JL. Cryptococcal meningitis in HIV negative pregnant women: case report and review of literature. Rev Inst Med Trop Sao Paulo. 2009;51(5):289–94.
44. Galgiani JN, Ampel NM, Blair JE, Catanzaro A, Johnson RH, Stevens DA, et al. Coccidioidomycosis. Clin Infect Dis. 2005;41(9):1217–23.
45. Bercovitch RS, Catanzaro A, Schwartz BS, Pappagianis D, Watts DH, Ampel NM. Coccidioidomycosis during pregnancy: a review and recommendations for management. Clin Infect Dis. 2011;53(4):363–8.
46. Walsh TJ, Anaissie EJ, Denning DW, Herbrecht R, Kontoyiannis DP, Marr KA, et al. Treatment of aspergillosis: clinical practice guidelines of the Infectious Diseases Society of America. Clin Infect Dis. 2008;46(3):327–60.
47. Perfect JR, Dismukes WE, Dromer F, Goldman DL, Graybill JR, Hamill RJ, et al. Clinical practice guidelines for the management of cryptococcal disease: 2010 update by the infectious diseases society of america. Clin Infect Dis. 2010;50(3):291–322.
48. Chapman SW, Dismukes WE, Proia LA, Bradsher RW, Pappas PG, Threlkeld MG, et al. Clinical practice guidelines for the management of blastomycosis: 2008 update by the Infectious Diseases Society of America. Clin Infect Dis. 2008;46(12):1801–12.
49. Pappas PG, Kauffman CA, Andes DR, Clancy CJ, Marr KA, Ostrosky-Zeichner L, et al. Clinical practice guideline for the management of candidiasis: 2016 update by the Infectious Diseases Society of America. Clin Infect Dis. 2016;62(4):e1–50.
50. Wheat LJ, Freifeld AG, Kleiman MB, Baddley JW, McKinsey DS, Loyd JE, et al. Clinical practice guidelines for the management of patients with histoplasmosis: 2007 update by the Infectious Diseases Society of America. Clin Infect Dis. 2007;45(7):807–25.
51. Kauffman CA, Bustamante B, Chapman SW, Pappas PG, Infectious Diseases Society of America. Clinical practice guidelines for the management of sporotrichosis: 2007 update by the Infectious Diseases Society of America. Clin Infect Dis. 2007;45(10):1255–65.

Chapter 7
Transfusion in Pregnant Patients Receiving Treatment for Leukemia

Mariângela Borges Ribeiro da Silva

7.1 Leukemia

Leukämie, a term used in German to describe an increase in leukocyte in peripheral blood, used to describe a clinical report of the first patient whose case was reported in 1845 by Rudolf Virchow, anatomical pathologist at the Charité Hospital of Berlin. This case was not the first to be reported, but it was the first described in a scientific way where it mentioned the first cellular transformations caused by the leukemic malignancy [1].

The first reported cases date from 1827 and were described by Velpeau [2].

Leukemia is a disease that comprises a group of malignant neoplasms that affect hematopoietic precursor cells.

Cellular disorder begins in the bone marrow, which produces hematological precursor cells, and subsequently the malignant cells overflow into the peripheral blood, thus reaching some organs and compromising the structure and activity of mature hematological cells [3].

The different types of leukemias have different causes, and they are involved in factors of DNA mutations due to genetic inheritance or environmental factors [4].

An important aspect of the biology of leukemia was the elucidation of the chromosomal spectrum and molecular mutations, as they cooperate in the pathways that lead to leukemogenesis. With the biotechnological tools developed, it is possible to describe the mutations associated with specific cytogenetic subsets of each type of leukemia [5–7].

Peter C. Nowell, from the University of Pennsylvania School of Medicine, and David Hungerford, from Fox Chase Cancer Center's Institute for Cancer Research, described, in 1960, the translocation between chromosome 9 and chromosome 22 (Philadelphia chromosome, Ph). This was the first gene described to cause cancer

M. B. R. da Silva (✉)
Uiversidade Federal do Paraná (UFPR), Curitiba, Brazil
e-mail: mariangela.borges@ufpr.br

© Springer Nature Switzerland AG 2021
C. W. P. Schmidt, K. M. Otoni (eds.), *Chemotherapy and Pharmacology for Leukemia in Pregnancy*, https://doi.org/10.1007/978-3-030-54058-6_7

and was extremely important in the development of the drug imatinib, the first medication with a genetic target [8, 9].

Since then, genetics has become of fundamental importance in the diagnosis, prognosis, and treatment of leukemias. Leukemias are prognostically determined by cytogenetic factors, more specifically acquired mutations that, once detected, enable the appropriate approach to the patient.

According to the cell of origin, leukemias can be classified into myeloid or lymphocytic, and according to the clinical behavior of the disease, leukemias can be classified into acute and chronic.

In this way, we have four main types of leukemias: acute lymphocytic leukemia (ALL), acute myelocytic leukemia (AML), chronic lymphocytic leukemia (LLC), and chronic myelocytic leukemia (CML) [10].

The US National Cancer Institute estimated that 61,780 people were diagnosed with leukemia in 2019. They were also able to predict that leukemia caused 22,840 deaths in the same year. Current data date back from 2016, thus for the year 2019, it is only possible to make forecasts because the information will be processed from some years from now. For the period from 2012 to 2016, 14.1 new cases were registered per year for every 100,000 inhabitants in the USA. In 2016, 414,773 people were diagnosed with leukemia in the USA. The most affected people were above the age of 55, but it is the most common cancer in children under 15 years of age [11].

Relative survival statistics compare the survival of patient's cancer diagnosed with the survival of people in the general population of the same age, race, and sex, who were not diagnosed with cancer. Since survival statistics are based on large groups of people, they cannot be used to predict exactly what will happen to a patient. No two patients are exactly alike, and treatment and responses to treatment can vary widely. However, the survival rate gives us information about the success of the treatment evolution of the disease.

In the mid-twentieth century, 100% of children with acute leukemia died, and medical intervention was considered by many to be inappropriate, useless, or unethical. Until a small number of pioneering scientists, like Sidney Farber and Donald Pinkel, changed this profile, and over several decades, the administration of combined drugs (antifolates, corticosteroids, and cytotoxic drugs) changed the international scenario and raised the rate of cure [12].

The survival rate increased from 33% in 1975 to 59% in 2005, and finally to 62.7% in 2015, and with promises to reach 90% with the new gene therapy treatments for the coming years [11].

Academic studies of leukemogenesis using animal models were fundamental for the development of antileukemic drugs. These include combined chemotherapy, stem cell transplantation, targeted monoclonal antibody therapy, and, more recently, gene therapy.

Monoclonal antibodies provided a crucial tool for the research and treatment of leukemia. First used to analyze and purify human cell populations, it was a product of immunological research, and, more recently, supported by Len Herzenber and collaborators, it has been used very efficiently in the treatment of several leukemia subtypes [13].

7.2   Leukemia and Pregnancy

The incidence of leukemia associated with pregnancy is extremely rare; it is estimated at 1 case for every 75,000 occurrences, and the acute forms are more frequent with almost 90% of the occurrences, and the remaining 10% are due to chronic leukemias, more commonly known as chronic myeloid leukemia [14].

Due to the severity of the disease, attention and interaction between obstetrician and hematologist are essential to guide the conduct when faced with this diagnosis.

Acute leukemias are difficult to manage in pregnancy. Treatment should be started immediately after diagnosis so that there is no harm to the maternal prognosis. Without treatment, the patient may die within months [15].

It is interesting that the diagnosis commonly occurs in the second and third trimesters of pregnancy, reducing the need for termination of pregnancy. However, when diagnosed in the first trimester, it is known that fetal losses will be greater in view of the chemotherapy to be employed [16].

The ethical dilemma created by the concomitance of neoplasms with pregnancy is difficult to manage. By promoting alternative treatments, with reduced risk of fetal impairment, maternal prognosis can be significantly altered [17].

The treatment of hematological neoplasms in pregnancy must consider the maternal risk and the consequences for the conceptual product, as well as the repercussions for the woman's reproductive future. For this, it is important that the performance of a multidisciplinary team with the participation of obstetricians, pediatricians, hematologists, and psychologists, who, together, must consider the stage and aggressiveness of the neoplasm, the gestational age, the associated maternal and fetal factors, as well as the preferences of the patient, in making decisions about the proposed conducts.

A problem that occurs frequently in this patient profile during pregnancy is the late identification of the diagnosis, since the initial symptoms of leukemia are camouflaged with the gestational symptoms. The treatment decision must consider the gestational phase and the fact of postpartum if necessary; to continue the treatment, the option of not breastfeeding must also be considered.

7.3   Therapeutic Apheresis

Even before blood transfusions to treat corrections of the leukemic patient's hematological profile, the blood bank can contribute to this treatment through a procedure performed by equipment—the automated blood cell separator, called therapeutic apheresis. This therapy is carried out with the purpose of removing an abnormal substance, or present in excess in the circulation, in the treatment of a certain disease. Apheresis is an adjunctive or complementary therapy. It cannot be used alone to treat the disease in question. Leukapheresis removes excess leukocytes and can be divided into removal of lymphocytes (lymphocyte apheresis), granulocytes (granulocyte apheresis), or the stimulated removal of hematopoietic progenitor cells (CPH—stem cells). The patient's hematologist makes the recommendation and the blood bank's hemotherapist assesses the possibility of the procedure and monitors and provides instructions.

For women in the chronic phase with leukocytosis and/or extreme thrombocytosis, leukapheresis is a possible alternative, mainly during the first and second trimesters, as it has the advantage of rapid reduction in counts without exposing the fetus to potentially teratogenic agents [18, 19].

Therapeutic apheresis has minimal risk for the fetus and pregnant woman. It should be used in cases where leukocytes are found in counts above 100×10^9/L and thrombocyte apheresis for platelet counts above 500×10^9/L [20].

7.4   Pharmacotherapeutic Treatment

7.4.1   Acute Leukemias

Drug therapy should be started as soon as the diagnosis has been made. Data demonstrate that survival was shown to be significantly longer in patients whose induction therapy was started before delivery than in those treated after delivery [21].

The risk of fetal injury induced by the administration of cytotoxic chemotherapy during the first trimester of pregnancy is real, even though it may occur in a minority of patients [22]. The development of new drugs with low teratogenicity has demonstrated efficacy in the treatment; however, for the current treatment regimen, it is still necessary to discuss the possibility of therapeutic abortion during the first trimester of pregnancy.

7.4.2   Acute Myeloid Leukemia

The treatment for acute leukemias goes through three phases: induction, consolidation, and maintenance. For the induction phase, the treatment of choice is anthracycline combined with cytarabine [23]; however, studies have shown that the combination of drugs increases fetal risks when compared to isolated drugs [24].

During the consolidation phase, high doses of cytarabine are administered; for this specific case of pregnancy, this phase must occur after delivery [23].

7.4.3 Acute Promyelocytic Leukemia

Treatment involves anthracycline combined with trans-retinoic acid [25].

7.5 Chronic Leukemias

7.5.1 Chronic Myeloid Leukemia

Pregnancy does not seem to affect the course of CML, and, sometimes, it does not require immediate treatment. However, the disease can increase the risk of placental insufficiency and the consequent low weight of the newborn, increasing rates of prematurity, morbidity, and perinatal mortality.

The conventional chemotherapy treatment for CML uses mainly the following components: hydroxyurea, busulfan (inhibitors of DNA synthesis) and interferon-alpha-2b, and a tyrosine kinase inhibitor called imatinib mesylate [26].

Despite the fact that imatinib has a potential teratogenic effect, case reports have been presented in the literature on the use of this drug in pregnancy without fetal involvement [17]. But still as a precaution, its use during pregnancy is not indicated.

7.5.2 Obstetric Considerations

Delivery should be planned at least 3 weeks after the last dose of chemotherapy to allow bone marrow recovery and minimize risks to the mother and fetus [27]. Chemotherapy should not be administered after 35 weeks due to immaturity of the liver and kidney; at this stage, neonates have limited capacity to metabolize and eliminate drugs. This time between chemotherapy and delivery will allow fetal drug excretion through the placenta [28].

7.6 Hemotherapeutic Support of Pregnant Women in Treatment of Leukemia

The basic indications for transfusions are to restore or maintain the oxygen transport capacity, blood volume, and hemostasis. The patient's clinical conditions, and not just laboratory results, are important factors in determining transfusion needs.

Despite all the surveillance, the transfusion procedure still presents risks (infectious disease, immunosuppression, alloimmunization) and should only be performed when there is a precise indication and no other therapeutic option.

As the transfusion procedure presents a potential risk, the decision must be shared by the medical team with the patient and family, and all doubts must be clarified. In situations related to religious beliefs, there are specific guidelines that should be discussed with the service's hemotherapist.

It is necessary for the patient to formalize the transfusion with the signing of a free and informed consent form that will clarify the transfusion procedure.

The participation of the hemotherapy service in the transfusion process is beneficial and will assist in some decision-making about the risks and benefits. Some guidelines are continually reviewed by the hemotherapy team, including the indication for transfusion. The transfusion request must be made exclusively by the attending physician and based on clinical criteria, and it will always be subjected to analysis by the physician at the hemotherapy service. Every transfusion carries risks, whether immediate or late, the benefits must outweigh the risks.

The request for the hemotherapy product must be filled out as completely as possible, prescribed and signed by a doctor, and be registered in the patient's medical record. There is no absolute contraindication to transfusion in patients with fever. It is important to decrease the fever before transfusion because the appearance of fever can be a sign of hemolysis or another type of transfusion reaction. No transfusion should exceed the 4-h infusion period. When this period has passed, the transfusion must be stopped and the unit discarded. No fluid or drug should be added to the blood product to be transfused. Red blood cell concentrates can be transfused in shared venous access only with 0.9% sodium chloride. It is unnecessary to dilute the red blood cell before the infusion. The hematocrit of the red cell concentrate generally allows a good flow of infusion. All blood products should be transfused with a 170 µm filter capable of retaining clots and aggregates.

7.7   Indication for Transfusion of Red Blood Cells

The transfusion of red blood cells (RBCs) should be performed to treat, or prevent, the imminent and inadequate release of oxygen to tissues.

Anemia should be corrected with packed red blood cells, and hemoglobin should be maintained above 7 g/dL.

Enough red blood cells should be transfused for the correction of hypoxia signs/symptoms or for Hb to reach acceptable levels. However, international committees defend the idea of increasing the safety of the transfusion process when the transfusion takes place with a single unit and the evaluation is carried out, and then the request for a new unit can be requested in sequence. In a medium-sized adult, transfusion of a red blood cells unit usually increases hematocrit by 3% and hemoglobin by 1 g/dL. The infusion time for each red blood cells unit should be 60–120 min in adult patients. The evaluation of the therapeutic response to red blood cells transfusion should be done through a new dose of hemoglobin or hematocrit 1–2 h after the transfusion, also considering the clinical response. In outpatients, laboratory evaluation can be done 30 min after the end of the transfusion and has comparable results [29].

7.8 Special Procedures in Blood Components for Transfusion in Immunosuppressed Patients

Some situations in the blood therapy clinic require additional care in the transfusion of blood components in hemato-oncological patients, including leukoreduction and irradiation.

7.8.1 Irradiation

Irradiation of blood components is performed to prevent transfusion-associated graft versus host disease (GVHD), a usually fatal immunological complication caused by grafting and clonal expansion of donor lymphocytes in susceptible recipients. In order to prevent this complication, cellular blood components (red blood cell and platelet concentrate) must be subjected to gamma irradiation at a dose of at least 2500 cGy (25 Gy), preventing the proliferation of lymphocytes. This procedure is indicated for patients with hematological diseases, recipient of any degree of kinship and human leukocyte antigen (HLA) compatible [30].

7.8.2 Deleucotization

It is a procedure performed through specific filters to remove leukocytes from a cellular blood component (red blood cells and platelets). One unit of whole blood contains about 2 to 3×10^9 leukocytes. The leukocyte component must contain less than 5×10^6 leukocytes. With this procedure, a 99% reduction in leukocytes occurs in a blood transfusion unit.

Most apheresis collection equipment already produces leukocyte blood components (leukocyte contamination less than 1×10^6 leukocytes). It is indicated in the prevention of complications related to the transfusion of allogeneic blood components due to the exposure of the recipient to the donor's leukocytes. This procedure is indicated for indications are contemplated pregnant women, and patients with leukemia [30].

The indication for this patient profile is to transfuse irradiated and leukoreduced blood components.

7.9 Erythrocyte Immunohematological Tests

Transfusion of red blood cell concentrate necessarily requires ABO and RhD compatibility. For this, pre-transfusion tests are performed to ensure compatibility between donor and recipient erythrocyte antigens.

Immunohematology is the study of antigens present on red blood cells (erythrocytes), the antibodies corresponding to them, and their clinical significance. The discovery of the first blood groups A, B, and O, in 1901, by the Austrian physician Karl Landsteiner, was the milestone between the empirical era and the scientific era in the history of hemotherapy. The beginning of the scientific era enabled the discovery of other blood group antigens, using the serological method to detect direct agglutination, resulting from the antigen-antibody reaction. In 1945, Coombs, Mourant, and Race described the Coombs test, preferably called the human antiglobulin test, one of the most important techniques used in the study of human blood groups. Human antiglobulin serum is used to detect antibodies that do not cause direct red blood cell agglutination, which revolutionized blood group serology, allowing the discovery of antibodies produced by alloimmunizations, resulting from transfusion or pregnancy. Currently, molecular biology has been responsible for another advance, with a special focus on the study of the structure and function of genetic material and its expression products, membrane proteins, which generate blood group antigens. Nowadays, more than 346 erythrocyte antigens have been described. Thus, it is necessary to know the compatibility between donor and recipient antigens and antibodies for a safe transfusion.

The quality of immunohematology in the execution of immunohematological tests—such as blood typing, compatibility test, research and identification of irregular antibodies, direct human antiglobulin test, and phenotyping—and the correct use of human antiglobulin serum is essential for the diagnosis of perinatal hemolytic disease, autoimmune hemolytic anemia, and transfusion management, contributing to transfusion safety.

In this case, ABO and RD tests are performed for donor and recipient and complementary tests such as: compatibility (crossmatch) tests and erythrocyte antibody testing in the patient's serum, in this specific case: female, young, pregnant patient, diagnosed with leukemia, and may be in chemotherapy treatment or not. The attention should be even greater because they are patients with a high possibility of presenting auto or alo antibodies due to the clinical state in which they present themselves. For transfusion safety in this case, if would be possible the patient must be phenotyped even before the start of chemotherapy treatment, thus ensuring the possibility of not forming any transfusion antibody.

These reports of information are extremely important to analyze the possibilities of results found in the tests performed pre-transfusion and thereby analyze the possible decision-making.

Some situations inherent to the profile of a pregnant patient with leukemia may interfere with pre-transfusion tests.

1. *Interferences by gene therapies*: There are still few reports of patients on gene therapies in large centers, especially patients diagnosed with leukemia and gestational status.
2. *Interferences by therapies with monoclonal antibodies*: Daratumumab anti-CD38 is a classic example; although it is not part of the treatment of leukemias, this monoclonal antibody brought us the first interference with erythrocyte antigens. It was the first concern with pre-transfusion tests, since the drug's mechanism of action targets molecules that are also erythrocyte antigens. The result was pan-reactivity in pre-transfusion tests. It brought us a warning signal for the mechanisms of action of new treatments. A new drug published in 2019 is the anti-CD47 Hu5F9-G4, used to treat refractory acute myeloid leukemia. This medication causes a decline in hemoglobin levels, and in pre-transfusion tests, there is pan-reactivity [31]. The hemotherapy service, for these cases, should be instructed to identify the patient's erythrocyte antigens and antibodies before starting treatment.
3. *Interference by chemotherapy therapies*: *Chemotherapy* drugs considerably decrease circulating antibodies; it is not common to see the discrepancy between antigen and antibody reactions in tests to identify ABO and Rh. In the absence of or reduction in antigens or antibodies, there are complementary temperature change techniques that can increase the sensitivity of the test. We can also change methodologies from tube to gel, increasing the sensitivity of the test. The discrepancy or identification of the antibody must be clarified before the transfusion process, for a correct and safe transfusion.
4. *Diagnostic interference—leukemia*: The chromosomal alterations caused by leukemia can alter the intensity of the expression of ABO and RhD antigens; during the phase of identification of these antigens, one must pay attention to the consensual evidence, to be sure of all the clarifications. In these cases, very rarely, it may be necessary to resort to DNA tests to complement the information for safe transfusion.
5. *Condition interference—pregnancy*: Pregnancy is a condition favorable to the development of all erythrocyte antibodies. When fetal erythrocytes come into contact with the maternal circulation, the damage can be harmful to both mother and fetus. There are reports of high-frequency antigen identified in this condition. For example, the antibody against high frequency antigen—anti-KANNO, is an antibody of clinical importance and pan-reactive. When antibodies against high-frequency antigen are developed, the possibility of finding a compatible donor becomes extremely rare. Monitoring is carried out by evaluating the search for irregular anti-erythrocyte antibodies [32].

7.10 Indication for Platelet Concentrate Transfusion

The platelet concentrate transfusion has drastically reduced death from hemorrhage in cases of AML. Basically, indications for unit platelet concentrate transfusion are associated with thrombocytopenia triggered by bone marrow failure.

Unit platelet concentrates contain approximately 5.5×10^{10} platelets in 50–60 mL of plasma, whereas apheresis units contain at least 3.0×10^{11} platelets in 200–300 mL of plasma (corresponding to 6–8 unit of random platet concentrat [33].

Platelet transfusion should be instituted when the count is less than 10,000/mm³ in a stable patient or less than 50,000/mm³ in a patient with bleeding or who needs an invasive procedure, which should be avoided because of both the hemorrhagic risk and the risk of bacterial circulation and sepsis. In addition to the number of platelets, the indication for transfusion should be considered in cases of mucosal bleeding, infection, severe mucositis, and fever [34].

Use platelets for transfusion collected by apheresis from single donors, preferably family members, for those cases whose bone marrow transplantation has been discarded but have compatible HLA. Studies report greater efficiency in transfusion of HLA-compatible platelet apheresis for immunocompromised patients. Blood components should be irradiated, given the risk of graft disease versus transfusion host.

7.11   ABO and RhD Compatibility of Platelet Concentrate

Platelets have ABO antigens on their surface, and levels of expression vary individually. There is evidence that transfusion of ABO incompatible reduces approximately 20% of increase in post-transfusion count, and seems to be more relevant when the natural antibody titers present in the receptor are highly associated with the high expression of the corresponding antigen in the platelets. This situation is uncommon. The clinical significance of incompatible ABO platelets transfusion seems to be of little relevance. In contrast, there is evidence that transfusion of ABO incompatible platelets develops refractoriness of immune cause—associated with alloimmunization—more often when compared to identical ABO platelet transfusions. In summary, transfusion of ABO compatible platelets should be preferred; however, if this is not possible, the option for transfusion of ABO incompatible units in patients who will not need chronic support. Alloimmunization against the RhD antigen is associated with contamination by red blood cells from platelets concentrate. Some studies demonstrate the occurrence of this alloimmunization in approximately 10% of RhD-negative patients transfused with positive RhD plateletes concentrate; it is more frequently in onco-hematological and pediatric patients because their exposure, and less frequently in those who receive platelets obtained by apheresis this cases that exposure is not be avoided its required using anti-D immunoprophylaxis (anti-D immunoglobulin) [35].

The recommended dose is 1 platelet concentrate unit for every 7–10 kg of the patient's weight, but the desired platelet count can also be considered, depending on the presence or absence of bleeding as follows: therapeutic transfusions (desired count greater than 40,000/µL): Adults > 55 kg in weight—minimum dose of 6.0 ×

10^{11} (8–10 U of CP unit or 1 U CP obtained by apheresis). Patients weighing 15–55 kg—minimum dose of 3.0×10^{11} (4–6 U unitary CP or 0.5–1 U CP obtained by apheresis). Smaller doses (1.5×10^{11} or 3–4 U of unitary CP) can be used in cases of prophylactic transfusions in stable patients without bleeding and maintained in a hospital with close monitoring. In this situation, the need for transfusion is more frequent, but it has been shown to be quite safe.

The infusion time of the CP dose should be approximately 30 min in adult or pediatric patients, not exceeding the infusion rate of 20–30 mL/kg/h. The evaluation of the therapeutic response to CP transfusion must be done through a new platelet count 1 h after the transfusion; however the clinical response must also be considered [36].

About 10% of pregnancies have maternal-fetal incompatibility, and 5% are at risk of alloimmunization. Data demonstrate that perinatal hemolytic disease has occurrence rates that vary from 1 to 6 occurrences for every 1000 cases.

7.12 Perinatal Hemolytic Disease (HDFN)

Disease of the fetus and newborn occurs due to the incompatibility of the blood group between an alloimmunized mother and the antigen-positive red blood cells of her fetus (inherited from the father). This condition was originally called hemolytic disease of the newborn because the condition (hemolysis and anemia) was seen in newborns or fetus. Untreated, progressing fetal anemia may result in hepatosplenomegaly, cardiomegaly, cardiac decompensation and eventually in fetal hydrops and perinatal death. If the fetus survives, persistent hemolysis may lead to severe neonatal hyperbili-rubinemia and brain injury, an irreversible condition known as 'kernicterus'. Women who have had multiple transfusions or are multiparous tend to form antibodies against blood group antigens. Antibodies associated with severe HDFN are mostly of the anti-Rh(D) type, and to a lesser extent of the anti-Kell (anti-K1) or anti-Rh(c) type. Severe HDFN is occasionally caused by other Rh-antibodies, and only very rarely by non-Rh antibodies (Duffy, Kidd, or S).

ABO incompatibility between a mother and her fetus is quite common, but HDFN for ABO incompatibility is clinically mild, mainly because ABO antigens are not fully expressed at birth, and anti-A and anti-B antibodies are predominantly of the immunoglobulin M (IgM) class. Antibodies directed against the RhD antigen can cause severe HDFN, and the fetus should be carefully monitored when the anti-D titer is greater than 16. With other blood group antibodies, the severity.

The indirect Coombs test thus makes it possible to determine whether, at some point, the mother produces antibodies against the fetus. Performed from a venous blood collection from the mother's forearm, it will detect the presence in the serum of anti erythrocyte antibodies that must be titrated and identified.

A positive result from the indirect Coombs test indicates isoimmunization (namely Rh incompatibility with the fetus); thus, antibodies against the fetal erythrocytes are in circulation, and the fetus may develop perinatal hemolytic disease. These cases require expert follow-up throughout pregnancy. Studies have found that administration of anti-D immunoglobulin (Ig) at 28 weeks of gestation in Rh-negative women is an effective intervention in the prevention of perinatal hemolytic disease, reducing the risk of isoimmunization from 2 to 0.1%.

In fetal or newborn hemolytic disease, it took time to recognize that dropsy, jaundice, and anemia were not three distinct conditions, but they were manifestations that reflect the severity of disease, and that the mothers of affected babies produced antibodies against the antigens from fetal blood groups absent in the mother but inherited from the father. This condition was initially called fetal erythroblastosis (meaning that the blood of a fetus contained erythroblasts), but it soon became known as newborn hemolytic disease, because the disease begins during pregnancy.

Hemolytic disease of the newborn (HDN) was first reported in a set of twins in 1609 by a French midwife. One was hydropic and still- born; the other became intensely jaundiced and died of kernicterus. The cause of hemolytic disease was determined by Levine [37]. Knowledge of (HDFN) in the 1940s when few blood groups were known (ABO, RhD) was restricted to the following: an affected baby was preceded by one or more unaffected babies, or by transfusion. Mothers of affected babies had severe reactions if transfused with their husbands' blood. Dr Bruce Chown, who founded the Rh Laboratory in 1944, in 1953 showed that the cause of Rh immunization was the passage of fetal Rh(D)- positive red cells into the maternal circulation [38]. Over 90% of mothers of babies with fetal erythroblastosis were RhD negative and their husbands were RhD positive, suggesting that anti-RhD was the identified antibody. However, about 10% of mothers with RhD positive were observed to have other major blood groups involved. Blood groups were not routinely determined, reagents were not available, and it was only possible to define which binding antibodies could be detected. Progress was made with the development of laboratory methods. No other immunohematology test with an impact on DHFN occurred until the 1990s, when erythrocyte genotyping was implemented. Progress also occurred with the advancement of methods for monitoring and treating the disease.

Anti-D antibodies used to be the most frequent immune antibodies, but with the introduction of RhD compatibility between donors and recipients in the late 1940s, as well as Rh immunoglobulin prophylaxis since the 1970s, their incidence has declined dramatically. Currently, anti-D is present in approximately 0.27–0.56% of transfusion recipients, 0.16–0.25% in blood donors, and 0.1–0.2% in pregnant women. In contrast, during the same period of time, the occurrence of immune antibodies against other antigens from blood groups has increased, although the actual absolute numbers are low. Other specificities besides anti-D are in approximately 0.6% of transfusion recipients, 0.19% of blood donors, and 0.14% of pregnant women.

There are several situations in which fetal red blood cells enter the maternal circulation and cause an immune response in the mother against the absent antigens. Some situations are childbirth, spontaneous bleeding, trauma, amniocentesis, cordocentesis, abortion, ectopic pregnancy, and chemotherapy treatments. If any of these events occur, Rh immunoglobulin should be administered.

The mother once alloimmunized, the more stimuli she receives, the higher the antibody titer. The maternal antibody (IgG) is carried through the placenta into the fetal circulation, where it binds to the corresponding antigen. IgG1 and IgG3 subclasses are more efficient than others in causing hemolysis; IgG1 is carried across the placenta earlier than IgG3 and in larger amounts. Fetal red blood cells attached to antibodies are recognized by Fc receptors in fetal macrophages, which lead to extravascular destruction in the spleen, causing progressive anemia and hyperbilirubinemia.

As the fetal red blood cells are destroyed, the hemoglobin released is broken down into nonconjugated (indirect) bilirubin, which passes into the maternal circulation and is conjugated with albumin in the maternal liver. Most antibodies cause this immune destruction of red blood cells in a hemolitic disease of newborn. However, certain antibodies, such as anti-K, anti-Kpa, and anti-Ge3 also inhibit erythropoiesis, leading to more severe anemia. Thus, it is important to identify the antibody when it is positive.

The fetus responds to anemia induced by increased red blood cell production, which leads to the presence of nucleated erythroid precursors in peripheral blood. As the anemia gets worse, the spleen and liver increase, and heart failure may occur. The liver decreases its production of albumin, which leads to decreased oncotic pressure, massive edema, ascites, and pleural and pericardial effusion; the most severe condition is called fetal hydrops. As bilirubin is usually conjugated by the maternal liver, the fetus is not icteric in utero. At birth, bilirubin cannot be efficiently metabolized by the immature fetal liver and remains in circulation of the newborn and can concentrate in the brain. When bilirubin levels are close to 25 mg/dL, irreversible brain damage, the so-called kernicterus, can occur. There is an increased risk of brain damage in a premature baby.

Currently, polymerase chain reaction (PCR) based assays are used to deduce an antigen from a blood group corresponding to the antibodies present in the maternal plasma. This is a genetic test to aid more accurate decision-making is particularly useful if the parent is heterozygous or not available for testing. If the fetus is positive for the antigen, the mother should be monitored, but if the fetus is negative for the antigen, there is no need to monitor the mother aggressively. When the father is heterozygous, fetal genotyping is of value in about 50% of pregnancies, and, as a result, invasive procedures are not necessary. When testing for a non-RhD antigen, it is always important to perform genotyping for the RHD gene. If an intrauterine transfusion is necessary, knowledge of this result may assist in the selection of the RBC concentrate.

Fetal DNA sources can be obtained from maternal plasma (after 12 weeks of pregnancy) or from amniocytes.

The conduct in (HDFN) is diverse and includes measures that must be taken when the fetus is still in the womb, as well as after birth.

Prenatal care includes checking the mother's history and performing basic immunohematological tests: determining the ABO and RhD blood groups of the mother and father and testing for antibodies in maternal plasma/serum are critical. Prenatal tests need to be performed on the mother's plasma/serum sample. If the antibody test is positive, the antibody(s) must be identified and the plasma/serum sample stored. The potential of an antibody to cause DHFN is usually determined by the effect the specificity of the antibody has had on other women. The antibody titer of the sample is determined and, if previous plasma/serum samples are available, they are tested in parallel and results are compared. Titers that potentially have clinical relevance are usually considered 16 for anti-D and only 2 for anti-K. Amniotic fluid can be tested for bilirubin levels, and fetal DNA can be tested to predict the blood group antigen(s) corresponding to the antibody(s) present in the maternal plasma. When an antibody with potential clinical significance is involved, the fetus should be monitored. If the fetus has signs of suffering, labor may be anticipated. To prevent the production of anti-RhD in non-alloimmunized RhD-negative women, it is recommended that Rh immunoglobulin be given at 28 weeks of gestation. Doppler ultrasound measures the peak velocity of fetal blood flow in the middle cerebral artery, is equivalent to the diagnosis of amniocentesis, but it has the advantage of not being invasive. It can be performed around the 18th week of gestation and correlates precisely with the severity of fetal anemia [39].

7.12.1 Intrauterine Transfusions

While the baby is still in the womb, a needle can be inserted into the umbilical vein (Doppler is used as a guide), thus providing direct access to the fetal circulation so that the transfused red blood cells circulate immediately in the fetus. In general, it is not performed before 20 weeks of gestation and with fetal hematocrit less than 30%. There is a 2% morbidity associated with each intrauterine transfusion procedure. Intrauterine transfusions can be repeated periodically until the 35th week, and delivery can be anticipated between the 37th and 38th week of gestation. Intrauterine transfusion, with each procedure, has an increased risk of alloimmunization and increased antibody titer. At the same time, a fetal blood sample can be obtained to determine ABO and RhD blood group, other relevant antigens, and hematocrit [39].

Phototherapy is the first step in the management of raised unconjugated jaundice in newborn infants. It is a safe and convenient method of lowering serum bilirubin levels and reduces the need for more invasive treatment, exchange transfusion. The predominant method of bilirubin elimination is the irreversible photoalteration of bilirubin to a structural which is a water-soluble compound and is excreted with bile and urine. The use of gestational age-specific treatment threshold graphs for babies with neonatal jaundice which is gestational age specific and gives a clear visual idea about the need for the modality of treatment at start as well as the response to treatment. High dose intravenous immunoglobulin is the only pharmacological treatment used in clinical practice for infants presenting with high jaundice levels secondary to rhesus or ABO isoimmunisation. Although it reduces the need for exchange transfusion, the duration of phototherapy and the length of hospital stay [40]. To prevent the production of anti-RhD in non-alloimmunized RhD-negative women, it is recommended that post-natal Rh immunoglobulin be administered within 72 h of birth.

7.12.2 Exchange Red Blood Transfusion

Exchange transfusion is more efficient at reducing bilirubin levels and is often used when maximal phototherapy and/or immunoglobulin are unsuccessful or when hemolysis is excessive but has known complications including vascular accidents, cardiovascular compromise, electrolyte and hematologic derangement. Furthermore, infants undergoing Exchange Transfusion are at higher risk of requiring intubation and mechanical ventilation, both of which are associated with additional complications. The parameters for decision making are when hyperbilirubinemia was defined as either a documented diagnosis of hyperbilirubinemia or a serum bilirubin level >15 mg/dL for infants 38 weeks gestation and older, or >10 mg/dL in infants aged ≤37 weeks prior to or on the day of Exchange transfusion, without evidence of an alternate diagnosis that may have justified a requirement for this. Atention for total bilirubin of 25 mg/dL or above is considered a medical emergency [41].

Whole blood or reconstituted whole blood is used to provide RBCs and clotting factors simultaneously. The procedure can be repeated if necessary. Recent or reconstituted whole blood can be used by group O (or ABO compatible), RhD negative, recent blood component (less than 7 days of storage), or, especially for rare blood, deglycerolized, AB plasma (fresh thawed and heated), a hematocrit ≥50% is desired, irradiated to prevent graft-versus-host disease, with serology negative for cytomegalovirus, concentrated RBCs should be leukoreduced.

References

1. Piller GJ. Leukaemia – a brief historical review from ancient times to 1950. Br J Haematol Hist Rev. 2001;112:282–92.
2. Ortiz-Hidalgo C. Notes on the history of leukemia. Patol Rev Latinoam. 2013;51:58–69.
3. Jahedi M, Shamsasenjan K, Sanaat Z, Aliparasti M, Almasi S, Mohamadian M, et al. Aberrant phenotype in Iranian patients with acute myeloid leukemia. Adv Pharm Bull. 2014;4(1):43.
4. Einollahi N, Alizadeh S, Dashti N, Nabatchian F, Zare Bovani M, Abbasi S, et al. Serum lipid profile alterations in acute leukemia before and after chemotherapy. Iran Blood Cancer J. 2013;6(1):3–9.
5. Carlson KM, Le Beau MM. Cytogenetics/fluorescent in situ hybridization. In: Young NS, Gerson SL, High KA, editors. Clinical hematology. Philadelphia: Elsevier; 2005. p. 1336–51.
6. Gilliland DG. Molecular genetics of human leukemias: new insights into therapy. Semin Hematol. 2002;39:6–11.
7. Shaffer LG, McGowan-Jordan J, Schmid C, editors. ISCN 2013: an international system for human cytogenetic nomenclature (2013). Recommendations of the International Standing Committee on Human Cytogenetic Nomenclature. Basel: S. Karger; 2013.
8. Nowell P, Hungerford D. A minute chromosome in human chronic granulocytic leukemia. Science. 1960;132:1497.
9. Nowell PC, Hungerford DA. Chromosome studies in human leukemia. II. Chronic granulocytic leukemia. J Natl Cancer Inst. 1961;27:1013–35.
10. Vardiman JW, Thiele J, Arber DA, Brunning RD, Borowitz MJ, Porwit A, Harris NL, Le Beau MM, Hellström-Lindberg E, Tefferi A, Bloomfield CD. The 2008 revision of the World Health Organization (WHO) classification of myeloid neoplasms and acute leukemia: rationale and important changes. Blood. 2009;114(5):937–51.
11. SEER. SEER stat fact sheets: leukemia: National Cancer Institute; 2019. https://seer.cancer.gov/statistics/
12. Pinkel D. A paediatrician's journey. In: Greaves M, editor. White blood: personal journeys with childhood leukaemia. Singapore/Hackensack: World Scientific; 2008. p. 13–46.
13. Herzenberg LA, et al. The history and future of the fluorescence activated cell sorter and flow cytometry: a view from Stanford. Clin Chem. 2002;48:1819–27.
14. Pavlidis NA. Coexistence of pregnancy and malignancy. Oncologist. 2002;7(4):279–87.
15. Rizack T, Mega A, Legare R, Castillo J. Management of hematological malignancies during pregnancy. Am J Hematol. 2009;84(12):830–41.
16. Chelghoum Y, Vey N, Raffoux E, Huguet F, Pigneux A, Witz B, et al. Acute leukemia during pregnancy: a report on 37 patients and a review of the literature. Cancer. 2005;104(1):110–7.
17. Ali R, Ozkalemkas F, Kimya Y, Koksal N, Ozkocaman V, Gulten T, et al. Imatinib use during pregnancy and breast feeding: a case report and review of the literature. Arch Gynecol Obstet. 2009;280(2):169–75.
18. Ali R, Ozkalemkaş F, Ozkocaman V, Ozçelik T, Ozan U, Kimya Y, Tunali A. Successful pregnancy and delivery in patient with CML and management of CML with leukapheresis during pregnancy. Jpn J Clin Oncol. 2004;34:215–7.
19. Klaasen R, de-Jong P, Wijermans PW. Successful management of chronic myeloid leukemia with leucapheresis during a twin pregnancy. Neth J Med. 2007;65:147–9.
20. Palani R, Milojkovic D, Apperley JF. Managing pregnancy in chronic myeloid leukaemia. Ann Hematol. 2015;94:167–76.
21. Kawamura S, Suzuki Y, Tamai Y, Itoh J, Fukushima K, Takami H. Pregnancy outcome among longterm survivors with acute leukemia. Int J Hematol. 1995;62:157–61.
22. Doll DC, Ringenberg S, Yarbro JW. Management of cancer during pregnancy. Arch Intern Med. 1988;148:2058–64.
23. Pagnano KBB, Rego EM, Rohr S, et al. Guidelines on the diagnosis na treatment for acute promyelocytic leukemia: Associação Brasileira de Hematologia, Hemoterapia e Terapia

Celular Guidelines. Project Associação Médica Brasileira 2013. Rev Bras Hematol Hemoter. 2014;36(1):71–92.

24. Koren G, Lishner M. Pregnancy and commonly used drugs in hematology practice. Hematology. 2010;2010:160–5.
25. Thomas X. Acute myeloid leukemia in the pregnant patient. Eur J Haematol. 2015;95(2):124–36.
26. Baccarani M, Saglio G, Goldman J, Hochhaus A, Simonsson B, Appelbaum F, et al. Evolving concepts in the management of chronic myeloid leukemia: recommendations from an expert panel on behalf of the European LeukemiaNet. Blood. 2006;108(6):1809–20.
27. Loibl S, von Minckwitz G, Gwyn K, et al. Breast carcinoma during pregnancy. International recommendations from an expert meeting. Cancer. 2006;106:237–46.
28. Sorosky JI, Sood AK, Buekers TE. The use of chemotherapeutic agents during pregnancy. Obstet Gynecol Clin N Am. 1997;24:591–9.
29. Carson JL, Guyatt G, Heddle NM, et al. Clinical practice guidelines from the AABB: Red blood cell transfusion thresholds and storage. JAMA. 2016;316(19):2025–35.
30. Fung MK, Grossman BJ, Hillyer CD, Westhoff C, editor. 18th ed. AABB. Technical manual; 2014.
31. Brierley CK, Staves J, Roberts C, Johnson H, Vyas P, Goodnough LT, Murphy MF. The effects of monoclonal anti-CD47 on RBCs, compatibility testing, and transfusion requirements in refractory acute myeloid leukemia. Transfusion. 2019;59(7):2248–54.
32. Kawabata K, Uchikawa M, Ohto H, Yasuda H, Tsuneyama H, Tsuchida H, Ito S. Anti-KANNO: a novel alloantibody against a red cell antigen of high frequency. Transfus Med Rev. 2014;28(1):23–8.
33. Roback JD, Grossman BJ, Harris T, Hillyer CD. AABB technical manual. 17th ed. Bethesda: American Association of Blood Banks; 2012.
34. Estcourt LJ, Birchall J, Allard S, Bassey SJ, Hersey P, Kerr JP, Mumford AD, Stanworth, SJ, Tinegate H. Guidelines for the use of platelet transfusions. Br J Haematol. 2017;176:365–394.
35. Villalba A, Santiago M, Freiria C, Montesinos P, Gomez I, Fuentes C, et al. Anti-D alloimmunization after RhD-positive platelet transfusion in RhD-negative women under 55 years diagnosed with acute leukemia: results of a retrospective study. Transfus Med Hemother. 2018;45(3):162–6.
36. Kaufman RM, Djulbegovic B, Gernsheime T, Kleinman S, et al. Platelet transfusion: a clinical practice guideline from the AABB. Ann Int Med. 2015;162(3):205–213.
37. Levine P, Katzin EM, Burnham L. Isoimmunization in pregnancy. JAMA. 1941;116(9):825.
38. Bruce C. Anæmia from bleeding of the fetus into the mother's circulation. The Lancet. 1954;263(6824):1213–15.
39. Nwogu LC, Moise KJ, Jr, Klein KL, Tint H, Castillo B, Bai Y. Successful management of severe red blood cell alloimmunization in pregnancy with a combination of therapeutic plasma exchange, intravenous immune globulin, and intrauterine transfusion. Transfusion, 2018;58:677–84.
40. Mitra S, Rennie J. Neonatal jaundice: aetiology, diagnosis and treatment. British J Hos. Med. 2017;78(12):699–704.
41. Wolf MF, Childers J, Gray KD, et al. Exchange transfusion safety and outcomes in neonatal hyperbilirubinemia. J Perinatol. 2020.

Chapter 8
Dose Adjustment of Chemotherapy for Leukemia in Pregnancy Based on Serum Dosages

Karla Rodrigues Andrade and Danilo Belchior Ponciano

Diagnosis of leukemia during pregnancy represents a major challenge for the patient, her family, and the medical and multidisciplinary team, as the optimal treatment may be associated with adverse effects on the fetus, including malformation and even death, which cause a significant maternal-fetal conflict. This dilemma becomes even more serious in the face of pregnancies where childbirth is not an option and patients do not have considerable time to make decisions, given the need to start treatment immediately [1].

Virtually, all drugs used in chemotherapy treatment of leukemia are category C or D according to the former US Food and Drug Administration system, indicating a lack of human studies, but there are animal studies suggesting adverse fetal effects (category C) or evidence of human fetal risk (category D). Changes in maternal physiology alter the bioavailability, distribution, clearance, and thus the half-life of the drug in often unpredictable ways. For most medications, pharmacokinetic and pharmacodynamic data in pregnancy are lacking. Some manufacturers suggest dose adjustments; however, current guidelines do not reflect these data [2].

As stated by Cardonick & Iacobucci, 2004, chemotherapy doses in pregnant patients are calculated based on the actual weight of patients with dose adjustment according to patients' weight gain during pregnancy. This seems coherent, since increased blood volume in pregnancy and increased renal clearance rate of medications can reduce the area under the curve and bioavailability of medications.

K. R. Andrade (✉)
Oncological Pharmaceutical Care Center at Hospital Sírio-Libanês, São Paulo, Brazil
e-mail: karla.r@andrade.pro.br

D. B. Ponciano
Bone Marrow Transplant Units of Hospital Sírio Libanês, São Paulo, Brazil

© Springer Nature Switzerland AG 2021
C. W. P. Schmidt, K. M. Otoni (eds.), *Chemotherapy and Pharmacology for Leukemia in Pregnancy*, https://doi.org/10.1007/978-3-030-54058-6_8

8.1   Acute Myeloid Leukemia

Given the poor quality of literature available [1], guidelines have been developed to standardize conducts and treatments that provide better care for patients with acute myeloid pregnant leukemia. Acute leukemias are the ones that affect pregnant women the most, with one-third of them being lymphoblastic and two-thirds myeloblastic [4].

When there is not enough time to induce labor, the standard chemotherapy regimen for acute myeloid leukemia (AML) (daunorubicin 60 mg/m^2 D1 D3 D5 and cytarabine 100 mg/m^2 Q 12h D1 to D10) is recommended [5]. This is a standard regimen in the UK. There are many anthracycline-based regimens known internationally, but there are no data to support the use of one specific regimen over the other [1]. Nevertheless, some studies support the use of higher doses of daunorubicin (90 mg/m^2 D1 D3 D5) [5] in AML patients, although this dose is not recommended for this group of patients. In short, the toxicity risk for pregnant patients undergoing these protocols is similar to the risk for nonpregnant patients. What frightens pregnant patients the most, however, is the risk of teratogenicity and fetal death [1].

According to FARHADFAR et al., 2017, patients with AML and PML were treated as follows: induction, idarubicin, and cytarabine; daunorubicin and cytarabine; idarubicin and cytarabine combined with nilotinib or all-trans retinoic acid (ATRA); daunorubicin and cytarabine in combination with thioguanine (6TG) or mercaptopurine (6MP).

8.2   Chronic Myeloid Leukemia

The incidence of chronic myeloid leukemia (CML) in pregnant women is 0.6 to 2 per 100,000 [7]. Occasionally, the diagnosis is an incidental finding during routine antenatal investigations [8]. The main therapeutic options available to CML patients during pregnancy are tyrosine kinase inhibitors, α-interferon, leukapheresis, and hydroxyurea [9].

Tyrosine kinase inhibitors (TKIs), such as imatinib, have become the first-line therapy for CML patients, promoting excellent response and improved life expectancy. The major challenge is the monitoring of pregnancies and the judicious use of specific target agents when seeking to reach a balance between the risk to mother's life and the harm to the fetus [9].

Pye et al. [10] argue that exposure to imatinib during pregnancy may result in an increased risk of serious fetal abnormalities or miscarriage and should be avoided in pregnant women unless discarding the therapy is considered unacceptable risk by the medical team. The risk/benefit assessment should be performed individually, with careful counseling to the parents, always seeking the latest data and alternative therapies. Information about risks of teratogenicity is limited in the literature regarding the use of dasatinib and nilotinib in pregnant women, and further studies are needed to establish their safety [11].

Alpha-interferon has been used to treat CML with variable performance. Its advantage over imatinib is that interferon does not cross the placental barrier due to its large molecular size, which minimizes the risk of teratogenicity and, therefore, reduces the risk of severe malformations, miscarriages, stillbirths, or premature births. However, it has significant neuropsychiatric, hematological, and hepatic sequelae that can severely affect the fetus's quality of life [12].

The use of hydroxyurea in pregnancy may result in minor fetal malformations, premature births, and preeclampsia, and there are no reports of improved survival for the mother [9].

Leukapheresis is an attractive short-term alternative therapy, especially for the first trimester, as it has not been shown to have adverse effects on the mother or fetus up to now [13].

8.3   Acute Lymphoid Leukemia

According to Farhadfar et al. [6], acute lymphoid leukemia (ALL) patients were treated with conventional therapy, which includes vincristine, doxorubicin, prednisone, cyclophosphamide, and L-asparaginase.

8.4   Monitoring

The risk of teratogenesis in humans is estimated to be lower than the risk normally observed in animals, as therapeutic doses used in humans are generally lower than the minimum teratogenic dose applied in animals. Exposure to chemotherapy in the first trimester has been associated with a 10–20% risk of severe malformation [14]. When using only one agent, this risk is even lower [15].

Most fetal malformations that occur after treatment with anthracyclines take place during the first trimester of pregnancy, especially when the exposure occurs between the 2nd and 8th weeks. In general, it is preferred to use daunorubicin or doxorubicin over idarubicin, for the last one is more lipophilic and favors placental transfer. There is much discussion about intrauterine exposure to anthracyclines, which are cardiotoxic to the fetus. However, it is established that serial prenatal ultrasound evaluation of fetal cardiac function plays an important role in the monitoring of cardiotoxicity or possible fetal heart failure [16]. Transient cardiomyopathy in neonates has been reported with idarubicin but not doxorubicin [3, 16] .

There is limited information on the use of cytarabine in pregnancy; however, the fact that it is an antimetabolite antineoplastic agent raises concern about its safe use and teratogenicity [17]. The risks are amplified when used in the first trimester, alone or in combination with other agents, presenting the following threats to the fetus: transnasal cytopenias, intrauterine fetal death, fetal growth restriction, and neonatal death secondary to sepsis [18, 19], even though the risk is relatively small.

Patients diagnosed with leukemia during pregnancy should be assisted by a specialized multidisciplinary team and be accompanied by a medical board consisting of oncohematologists, obstetricians, anesthetists, and neonatologists. The health of the mother and the baby must always be taken into account, and the informed wishes of the mother, who should always be informed about the diagnosis, treatment, and possible complications, must be honored [1].

Pregnant women with a leukemia diagnosis and undergoing chemotherapy should receive regular obstetric hematological examination with biweekly ultrasound scans to detect fetal growth restrictions and assess fetal well-being [1].

References

1. Ali S, et al. Guidelines for the diagnosis and management of acute myeloid leukaemia in pregnancy. Br J Haematol. 2015;170(4):487–95.
2. Ansari J, Carvalho B, Shafer SL, Flood P. Pharmacokinetics and pharmacodynamics of drugs commonly used in pregnancy and parturition. Anesth Analg. 2016;122(3):786–804. https://doi.org/10.1213/ane.0000000000001143.
3. Cardonick E, Iacobucci A. Use of chemotherapy during human pregnancy. Lancet Oncol. 2004;5:283–91.
4. Hurley TJ, McKinnel JV, Irani MS. Hematologic malignancies in pregnancy. Obstet Gynecol Clin North Am. 2005;32:595–614.
5. Burnett AK, et al. A randomized comparison of daunorubicin 90 mg/m2 vs 60 mg/m2 in AML induction: results from the UK NCRI AML17 trial in 1206 patients. Blood. 2015;125(25):3878–85.
6. Farhadfar N, et al. Acute leukemia in pregnancy: a single institution experience with 23 patients. Leuk Lymphoma. 2017;58(5):1052–60.
7. Tadwalkar S. The global incidence and prevalence of chronic myeloid leukemia over the next ten years (2017–2027). J Blood Disord Transfus. 2017;8:2.
8. Apperley J. Issues of imatinib and pregnancy outcome. J Natl Compr Cancer Netw. 2009;7(10):1050–8.
9. SAMAL R, et al. Chronic myeloid leukaemia in pregnancy: call for guidelines. J Obstet Gynaecol J Inst Obstet Gynaecol. 2019;39(4):582–3.
10. Pye SM, Cortes J, Ault P, Hatfield A, Kantarjian H, Pilot R, et al. The effects of imatinib on pregnancy outcome. Blood. 2008;111:5505–8.
11. Barkoulas T, Hall PD. Experience with dasatinib and nilotinib use in pregnancy. J Oncol Pharm Pract. 2018;24(2):121–8.
12. Yazdani Brojeni P, Matok I, Garcia Bournissen F, Koren G. A systematic review of the fetal safety of interferon alpha. Reprod Toxicol (Elmsford, New York). 2012;33:265–8.
13. Bhandari A, Rolen K, Shah BK. Management of chronic myelogenous leukemia in pregnancy. Anticancer Res. 2015;35(1):1–11.
14. Weisz B, Meirow D, Schiff E, Lishner M. Impact and treatment of cancer during pregnancy. Expert Rev Anticancer Ther. 2004;4:889–902.
15. Doll DC, Ringenberg QS, Yarbro JW. Management of cancer during pregnancy. Arch Intern Med. 1988;148:2058–64.

16. Meyer-Wittkopf M, Barth H, Emons G, Schmidt S. Fetal cardiac effects of doxorubicin therapy for carcinoma of the breast during pregnancy: case report and review of the literature. Ultrasound Obstet Gynecol. 2001;18:62–6.
17. Shapira T, Pereg D, Lishner M. How I treat acute and chronic leukemia in pregnancy. Blood Rev. 2008;22:247–59.
18. Cantini E, Yanes B. Acute myelogenous leukemia in pregnancy. South Med J. 1984;77:1050–2.
19. Aviles A, Niz J. Long-term follow-up of children born to mothers with acute leukemia during pregnancy. Med Pediatr Oncol. 1988;16:3.

Chapter 9
Supportive Drugs in Leukemia Treatment During Pregnancy

Celina de Jesus Guimarães, Sarah Sant' Anna Maranhão,
Pedro Mikael da Silva Costa, and Claudia Pessoa

9.1 Introduction

The diagnosis of cancer during pregnancy is uncommon. Breast, melanoma, and cervical cancers are those most diagnosed during pregnancy, followed by hematological malignancies [1]. Hematological malignancies are diseases that generally affect the bone marrow and cause impaired hematopoiesis and require special attention for their complications.

Despite advances in the treatment of leukemia, which have prolonged survival and even made cure possible in many instances, the low incidence of leukemia occurring during pregnancy and possibly the under-reporting of cases have adversely affected the understanding of managing such cases [2]. The incidence of leukemia associated with pregnancy is estimated to be 1 in 10,000 pregnancies [3].

The coincidence in the occurrence of leukemia during pregnancy leads to a dilemma to the patient, the hematologist, and the obstetrician in terms of the usage of cytotoxic agents with potential adverse effects, which require supportive treatment and multidisciplinary team approach [3].

The principles for leukemia therapy during pregnancy are the same applied to non-pregnant patients and cause doubts regarding the risks for the mother and the fetus [4]. However, supportive therapy choice must consider the risks and benefits during pregnancy, considering that clinical studies have not been conducted in this population. Pregnant females or mothers with terminated pregnancies due to

C. de Jesus Guimarães (✉)
Laboratory of Experimental Oncology, Research and Development of Medicines Center, Universidade Federal do Ceará, Fortaleza, Brazil

Fundação Centro de Controle de Oncologia do Estado do Amazonas, Manaus, Brazil

S. S. A. Maranhão · P. M. da Silva Costa · C. Pessoa
Laboratory of Experimental Oncology, Research and Development of Medicines Center, Universidade Federal do Ceará, Fortaleza, Brazil
e-mail: cpessoa@ufc.br

© Springer Nature Switzerland AG 2021
C. W. P. Schmidt, K. M. Otoni (eds.), *Chemotherapy and Pharmacology for Leukemia in Pregnancy*, https://doi.org/10.1007/978-3-030-54058-6_9

145

cytotoxic chemotherapy treatment require supportive care with fluids for hydration and nutritional supplements, safe antimicrobials to treat various infectious complications, growth factors to shorten the periods of neutropenia and blood product transfusions as needed [5].

Indeed, induction chemotherapy in pregnant women with leukemia is an option restricted to the second and third trimesters. Usually, the strategies are combining anthracyclines and cytarabine, for acute myeloid leukemia (AML), or use of all-trans-retinoic acid for acute promyelocytic leukemia. Treatment protocols in adult acute lymphocytic leukemia (ALL) are typically risk-adapted, using a combination of vinca alkaloids and corticosteroids with anthracyclines. In case of patients with Philadelphia-positive ALL, imatinib mesylate is added to chemotherapy [4].

Chemotherapy often results in adverse events, including nausea, infections, anemia, hemorrhages, allergy reactions, and others, and using a combination of all of these during leukemia treatment can induce severe pancytopenia, infections, nausea, vomiting, and require adequate supportive care [5]. Neutropenia, for example, entails a considerable risk of infection and may require intravenous broad-spectrum antibiotics and antifungal treatment. Just as patients with anemia require transfusions, so does thrombocytopenia to prevent or treat bleeding [4].

Supportive drugs generally used for management of adverse events in relation to chemotherapy, such as selective bowel decontamination like quinolones or sulfonamides, several antibiotics for intravenous use, antihistaminic antacids, certain analgesic drugs and other compounds are contraindicated or not advisable during pregnancy [6].

When it comes to pregnancy, the US Food and Drug administration (FDA) established five-letter risk categories—A, B, C, D, and X—that indicate the potential of a drug to cause any harm to the fetus during pregnancy. The drugs are categorized based on reliable documents that determine the risk to benefit ratio (Table 9.1).

Essential points relate to the provision of the best treatment to achieve cure or a good survival rate of the mother and to minimize the related toxic effects to the fetus [8]. This has led to a rise in such cases due to older age for pregnancy, especially in developed countries, showing the urgent need for strict guidelines about the theme [9].

9.2 Symptoms the Supportive Treatment in Leukemia

9.2.1 Nausea and Vomiting

Nausea and vomiting are frequent symptoms in pregnancy, affecting up to 80% of all pregnancies, and also the most serious side effects of chemotherapy [10]. When combined together, these events require special care and attention. Chemotherapy-induced nausea and vomiting (CINV) may cause malnourishment and consequently affect the immune system, electrolyte imbalance, and quality of life. These kinds of

Table 9.1 Categories of drugs for use in pregnancy

Category	FDA definition
A	Adequate and well-controlled studies in pregnant women have failed to demonstrate a risk to the fetus in the first trimester of pregnancy.
B	Animal reproduction studies have failed to demonstrate a risk to the fetus, but there are no adequate and well-controlled studies of pregnant women. Or animal studies demonstrate a risk, and adequate and well-controlled studies in pregnant women have not been conducted during the first trimester.
C	Animal reproduction studies have shown an adverse effect on the fetus, but there are no adequate and well-controlled studies of humans. The benefits from the use of the drug in pregnant women might be acceptable despite its potential risks. Or animal studies have not been conducted, and there are no adequate and well-controlled studies of humans.
D	There is positive evidence of human fetal risk based on adverse reaction data from investigational or marketing experience or studies of humans, but the potential benefits from the use of the drug in pregnant women might be acceptable despite its potential risks.
X	Studies in animals or humans have demonstrated fetal abnormalities, or there is positive evidence of fetal risk based on adverse reaction reports from investigational or marketing experience, or both. The risk involved in the use of the drug in pregnant women clearly outweighs any possible benefits.

Source: From FDA [7]

side effects can lead to a reduction in cure related to treatment interruption or chemotherapy dose reduction [11].

Chemotherapy emesis is classified into four groups: minimally emetogenic chemotherapy, in which emesis occurrence is less than 10% and includes drugs such as bevacizumab, vinorelbine, bleomycin, nivolumab, rituximab, and vincristine. Low emetogenic chemotherapy, in which emesis occurrence is between 10% and 30% and includes drugs such as fluorouracil, docetaxel, and trastuzumab. Moderately emetogenic chemotherapy, with the emesis occurrence between 30% and 90% and includes regimens with carboplatin, irinotecan, oxaliplatin, and etoposide. High emetogenic chemotherapy, in which the emesis occurrence is greater than 90% and includes regimens with cisplatin, doxorubicin plus cyclophosphamide, dacarbazine and epirubicin plus cyclophosphamide [12, 13]. Based on this classification, patients who are undergoing treatment for chronic myeloid leukemia (CML) receiving imatinib usually have less CINV than patients undergoing treatment for non-Hodgkin lymphomas (NHL) and acute myeloid leukemia (AML), who are being treated with doxorubicin.

Physiologic pathways involved in CINV are not completely elucidated but a number of neuroreceptors have been identified and include serotonin, neurokinin-1, and dopamine as the main players in the treatment of emesis. Other receptors can also be involved in these processes and include cholinergics, corticosteroids, histamine, cannabinoid, and opioid receptors [14, 15]. Antiemetic therapy for chemotherapy-induced nausea and vomiting includes various treatments with serotonin receptor antagonists, dopamine receptor antagonists, neurokin-1 receptor antagonists, vitamin B6, metoclopramide, and natural options such as ginger.

5-HT$_3$ Receptor Antagonists

The 5-HT$_3$ receptor antagonist was the first class of agents developed specifically for antiemesis. Selective serotonin receptor antagonists block serotonin both on vagal nerve terminals in the gastrointestinal system and centrally in the chemoreceptor trigger zone in the postrema area, resulting in very effective antiemetics [15, 16]. Usually, prophylaxis for highly emetogenic chemotherapy regimens comprises serotonin type 3 (5-HT$_3$) receptor antagonists that include palonosetron, ondansetron, and granisetron in combination with dexamethasone [17].

Ondansetron is a first-generation 5-HT$_3$ receptor antagonist with a low cost. Ondansetron showed in different studies a similar efficacy than granisetron and tropisetron for CINV [18]. But when it comes to pregnancy, ondansetron was classified as Pregnancy Category B by Food and drug administration (FDA). Despite that, ondansetron is widely used across the United States for both nausea and vomiting during pregnancy as an oral antiemetic [19]. Lavecchia and coworkers showed the lack of evidence linking prenatal exposure to ondansetron to an increased risk of congenital malformations in a systematic review. There is still a need for additional epidemiologic studies to confirm whether ondansetron represents a safe alternative treatment for nausea and vomiting in pregnancy [20].

Granisetron is another 5-HT$_3$ receptor antagonist that is FDA approved for the treatment of CINV comparable to ondansetron. Granisetron can be administered via intravenous or a transdermal patch, offering an alternative option to those pregnant women with severe signs and symptoms of nausea and hyperemesis. A study performed in 2016 recruited 15 pregnant women for IV administration and 13 pregnant women for patch placement between 12 and 18 weeks' gestation. Granisetron significantly improved symptoms of nausea and vomiting, but no data about fetus safety were analyzed [21].

Another study performed in 2019 compared patient's newborn health who received the drug to those who did not receive the drug based on a detailed health questionnaire. Authors concluded that exposure to granisetron in early pregnancy is not associated with adverse fetal/neonatal outcomes and provides preliminary reassurance regarding the safety of in utero exposure to granisetron [22].

Palonosetron is a second-generation 5-HT$_3$ receptor antagonist indicated for the prevention of acute and delayed nausea and vomiting. It is distinguished from other 5-HT$_3$ receptor antagonists by the prolonged half-life, high binding affinity, and better efficacy than the first-generation 5-HT$_3$ receptor antagonists such as ondansetron and dolasetron [17, 23]. There is a lack of studies about the use of palonosetron in pregnant women. Akynzeo (netupitant plus palonosetron) is listed as pregnancy category C, but there are no adequate and well-controlled studies with these drugs in pregnant women [24].

Neurokinin 1-Receptor Antagonists

Neurokinin-1 (NK$_1$) receptors are involved with delayed CINV, and the process is mediated by substance P. Endogenous substance P binds with high affinity to the NK$_1$ receptors localized in the central nervous system (CNS), which then transfer the signal to the chemoreceptor trigger zone (CTZ) and the vomiting center (VC).

NK$_1$ receptor antagonists act by blocking the binding of substance P, avoiding the activation of the brain-stem emetic center. NK$_1$ receptor antagonists approved for prevention of CINV include aprepitant, rolapitant, and netupitant [14].

In case of chemotherapy of high emetic risk, NK$_1$ receptor antagonists are combined with 5-HT$_3$ receptor antagonist plus dexamethasone [13, 25]. In pregnancy, there are no controlled data related to direct or indirect harm for fetal development for this antiemetic class. Rolapitant was tested in animal reproduction studies, and there were no teratogenic or embryo-fetal effects observed with oral administration in rats and rabbits (doses up to 1.2 times and 2.9 times the maximum recommended human dose, respectively). FDA data inform that in US general population, the risks of major birth defects and miscarriage in clinically recognized pregnancies is 2–4% and 15–20%, respectively. FDA has classified NK$_1$ receptor antagonists as category B for pregnancy classification.

Dopamine receptor Antagonists

Dopamine is a neurotransmitter that plays several crucial roles in brain, including nausea and vomiting. There are five different subtypes of dopamine receptors (D1–D5). However, the two most prevalent dopamine receptors in the brain are D1 and D2. D2 receptor subtypes are located in the CTZ and are stimulated by the gastrointestinal (GI) tract, being an effective pharmacological target for treating nausea and vomiting [26]. Dopamine receptor antagonists such as metoclopramide may be considered for prophylaxis in patients with low emetic risk, who are receiving chemotherapy [12].

Metoclopramide acts both centrally in the brain and peripherally in the GI system, blocking D2 and 5-HT$_3$ receptors. Due to the ability to cross blood-brain barrier, the drug causes extrapyramidal side effects [15]. Metoclopramide may be administered orally or intravenously, and the usual dose is 10–20 mg. During pregnancy, metoclopramide use was not associated with increased risk of major congenital malformations or evidence of increased risk for adverse pregnancy, fetal or neonatal outcomes [27–31]. A published study comparing the effectiveness of ondansetron and metoclopramide in severe nausea and vomiting in pregnant women showed that the 5-HT$_3$ receptor antagonist had more favorable effect in controlling severe vomiting when compared to metoclopramide [32].

Bromopride is another dopamine antagonist used as an antiemetic agent. Bromopride is the bromo analog of metoclopramide, usually used to treat gastric motility dysfunction, nausea, and vomiting. The most serious side effects described are extrapyramidal reactions. In Brazil, the use of bromopride is well tolerated and quite widespread, but in the United States the drug is not available [33]. Bromopride is not commonly used for the treatment of CINV, since when compared to ondansetron, it had an inferior antiemetic effect [34]. The use of bromopride during pregnancy appears to be safe and effective, but there are few studies in humans proving this statement [35]. It is necessary more data related to fetus safety for bromopride use.

Alternative Antiemetics for Pregnancy

There are alternative antiemetic safe drugs that can be used during pregnancy, but they are not an elective treatment for CINV. Ginger, pyridoxine, and antihistamines were associated with greater benefit to treat mild symptoms of nausea and emesis during pregnancy. In case of moderate symptoms, the use of doxylamine/pyridoxine and ondansetron was associated with improved symptoms compared with placebo [30].

Dimenhydrinate is an antihistamine and anticholinergic that acts in the brain. Dimenhydrinate is a Category B drug for pregnancy classified by FDA and can be associated with pyridoxine (vitamin B6). Vitamin B6, a water-soluble vitamin essential in the folate metabolism pathway, is a first-line treatment for nausea and vomiting during pregnancy and belongs to FDA pregnancy category A. The pyridoxine mechanism in the treatment of nausea is unknown. When compared separately, dimenhydrinate was more effective than vitamin B6 when tested in 135 women pregnant with a gestational age of < 16 weeks [36].

Pyridoxine can also be combined with doxylamine, a first-generation antihistamine. The use of this combination is licensed for the treatment of nausea and vomiting during pregnancy when first-line treatment has not worked [37]. A randomized, double-blind, multicenter placebo-controlled trial showed that the drug combination was effective and well tolerated in the treatment of nausea and vomiting during pregnancy when compared to placebo [38]. Common adverse effects related to doxylamine are sedative and hypnotic effects, factors that decrease the drug use.

Ginger (*Zingiber officinale*) is a nonpharmacological treatment for nausea and vomiting during pregnancy. Ginger showed to be as effective as dimenhydrinate and pyridoxine in the treatment of nausea and vomiting and has fewer side effects [39–42]. Cohort safety studies were conducted in women in the first or second trimester, finding no associations between the use of ginger and malformations, stillbirth, or spontaneous abortion [43, 44]. However, Choi and coworkers showed in a small study ($n = 441$) that was a trend of increased stillbirths and major malformation after ginger use [45]. Based on that clinical evidence, ginger is contraindicated close to labor or in those with a history of miscarriage [46].

9.2.2   Hemorrhages and Thrombosis

It is well recognized that cancer patients have an increased risk of thrombosis and bleeding. The incidence of thrombosis in a cancer patient is 30% higher than the general population and is even higher in those with hematological malignancies [47]. Patients with B-cell malignancies have an increased risk of bleeding, especially patients with Mantle cell lymphoma and chronic lymphocytic leukemia who are at an approximately eight-fold increased risk of major hemorrhages in comparison to the age- and sex-matched general population [48]. Adverse hemorrhagic events are related to hematological malignancies and represent a major cause of morbidity and mortality [49].

Many contributory factors account for the increased risk for thrombosis such as chemotherapeutic agents, type of cancer, stage of cancer, age, and comorbidities. In patients with acute lymphoblastic leukemia (ALL), one of the main risk factors for the development of venous thromboembolism (VTE) has been the use of L-asparaginase. Patients with acute promyelocytic leukemia have high risk of VTE and bleeding. Patients with aggressive lymphomas have a high risk of VTE. Meanwhile, patients with multiple myeloma are at highest risk of VTE in those who receive immunomodulatory agents such as thalidomide or lenalidomide. Another important point is thrombocytopenia.

Thrombocytopenia in hematologic malignancies is not only therapy related but can also be associated with disease infiltration in bone marrow, ablation from stem cell transplant conditioning and immune mediated. Therefore, treatment of VTE in patients who have a hematologic malignancy is more complex than for solid tumors, requiring pharmacologic prevention and treatment of VTE [50].

Tranexamic Acid
Tranexamic acid (TA)—(trans-4-(aminomethyl) cyclohexane-carboxylic acid)—is a synthetic derivative of the amino acid lysine that binds to kringle domains and inhibits the activation of plasminogen. TA blocks the lysine-binding sites of plasminogen, resulting in inhibition of plasminogen activation and fibrin binding to plasminogen [51]. Thus, TA also impairs fibrinolysis. Several clinical trials proved the efficacy of TA administration, reducing traumatic bleeding [52], surgical bleeding [53, 54], and post-partum hemorrhage [55, 56]. A study conducted by Ducloy et al. showed that the use of high-dose TA (4 g over 1 h) decreased bleeding duration and made the progression to severe post-partum hemorrhage less frequent [57]. The appropriate dose, indication, and duration of TA remain unknown. TA is an FDA pregnancy category B, but since TA is effective in the prevention and management of bleeding during pregnancy, it seems to be safe [58]. However, it is still uncertain whether TA may be associated with an increased risk of arterial and venous thromboembolism [51].

Vitamin K Supplementation
Vitamin K, a fat-soluble vitamin, is a necessary co-factor for the activation of factors II, VII, IX, X, and proteins C and S. Vitamin K administration is usually prescribed when clinical deficiencies are detected or following routine investigation [59]. During pregnancy, vitamin K can present a serious health risk linked to hemorrhage. Vitamin K deficiency is extremely rare among the general adult population but can be increased in women who ingest anticonvulsants such as warfarin and heparin, and antibiotics such as cephalosporin. There is insufficient evidence to show that excessive vitamin K ingestion is related to toxic effects, but it passes through the placenta and is found in breast milk. Therefore, pregnant and lactating women should look for advice from their health practitioner [60, 61]. An old double-blind study warned the association between vitamin K administration and neonatal hyperbilirubinemia [62].

Heparins

Heparin and low-molecular-weight heparin (LMWH) are administered as a veno-occlusive disease prophylaxis. Treatment of VTE in patients who have a hematological malignancy is preferably with heparin than warfarin [50]. Heparin is a naturally occurring polysaccharide that inhibits coagulation. Heparin works by binding antithrombin and thrombin, producing an effect on thrombin and factor X. Heparin advantage is related to its fast action added to a short half-life with an instantaneous action stop. An important heparin adverse effect is the heparin-induced thrombocytopenia (HIT). HIT can occur in up to 5% of patients, and it is characterized by a reduction in platelet count > 50% from baseline prior to heparin, hypercoagulability, and heparin-dependent platelet-activating immunoglobulin antibodies [63]. Non-fractionated heparin usually is not administered to pregnant women since it is classified as FDA Pregnancy Category C even if it is not able to cross the placenta and is not excreted in human milk. During pregnancy, low-molecular-weight heparins are the first-line treatment for VTE.

Enoxaparin

Low-molecular-weight heparins (LMWHs) have shorter polysaccharide chains and lower molecular weights than unfractionated heparins. LMWHs are widely used mainly for thromboprophylaxis and are usually administered subcutaneously [64]. LMWH principal effector is factor Xa with less inhibitory activity against thrombin (factor IIa). The incidence of HIT for LMWH is lower than 1% [63]. Enoxaparin is a very popular LMWH widely used during pregnancy [65] and VTE related to hematological malignancies [66, 67]. Systematic review and meta-analysis studies showed that the exposure to enoxaparin during pregnancy was not associated to increased risk of teratogenicity and other major malformations in general, and there was a significantly lower occurrence of pregnancy loss [65, 68, 69].

Desmopressin

Desmopressin acetate (DDAVP) is a synthetic analogue (1-deamino-8-D-argenine vasopressin) of the antidiuretic hormone L-arginine-vasopressin. DDAVP stimulates the export of von Willebrand factor (VWF) from storage organelles, and von Willebrand factor acts by increasing the adhesion of platelets to the subendothelium. DDAVP is found to be an effective drug, which can reduce the risk of hemorrhages, especially in patients with acquired von Willebrand syndrome [70]. In patients with bleeding disorders, DDAVP infusion results in a two- to six-fold increase from baseline in factor VII and VWF plasma levels, although individuals have differing responses, with a pick level in 30–90 min. DDAVP is an FDA Pregnancy Category B and seems to be safe for the fetus since it does not cross the placenta, and it does not pass into breast milk in any significant amount [71, 72].

Blood Components

Blood components can be used as a systematic therapy of bleeding in patients with hematologic malignancies and usually consist of platelets, fresh frozen plasm, coagulation factors concentrate, cryoprecipitates, single factors (FVII, FVIII, FIX, von Willebrand factor) administration, and immunoglobulin. All the nonpharmacological blood components cited can be used during pregnancy and must be followed closely by the clinicians [70, 73].

Warfarin

Warfarin is a vitamin K antagonist, which prevents the production of clotting factors, blocking regulatory anticoagulant proteins (proteins C, S, and Z) and factors II, VII, IX, and X. Warfarin remains the most utilized anticoagulant in the treatment of VTE among cancer patients [63]. When it comes to hematological malignancies, low-molecular-weight heparins are preferred to warfarin because they are more effective than warfarin [74] and can be associated with the impairment of bone marrow microenvironment and hematopoiesis [75]. Warfarin is FDA Pregnancy Category D, and the use should be avoided during pregnancy, especially during the first trimester because of teratogenicity. Between 6 and 12 weeks' gestation, fetal synthesis of proteins crucial for bone and cartilage formation may be impaired by warfarin, resulting in the defined "warfarin embryopathy" [76, 77]. Use at any point during pregnancy may increase the risk of fetal intracranial hemorrhage and schizencephaly [78].

9.2.3 Tumor Lysis Syndrome

Tumor lysis syndrome (TLS) is a medical condition characterized by rapid onset of hyperuricemia, hyperkalemia, hypokalemia, hyperphosphatemia, and renal impairment. The cause of TLS is the rapid release of intracytoplasmic components during cellular lysis that may follow the initiation of cancer therapy, or it can occur spontaneously. TLS is a potentially life-threatening condition usually associated with hematological malignancies, particularly acute leukemias and non-Hodgkin lymphomas, being less frequent in solid cancers [79].

Different risk factors can be pointed out for the occurrence of TLS such as type of cancer, tumor burden, hyperleukocytosis, metastasis, and other important clinical findings. Further, concomitant patient conditions such as kidney functions, metabolic dysfunction, and hydration level can also play a role during TLS. For example, high proliferative diseases as Burkitt's lymphoma (BL) or acute lymphoblastic leukemia (ALL) are often more chemosensitive [80].

TLS patients have biochemical abnormal features with or without clinical manifestation; in both cases, treatment management is required. Laboratory features related to TLS include abnormality of two or more of the following: uric acid, potassium, phosphorus, and calcium. Several symptoms may appear due to TLS, including renal, cardiac, neurological, and muscular manifestations [81]. TLS prevention and management are recommended to all patients with hematological malignancies undergoing chemotherapy and consist of hydration, use of drugs that decrease uric acid (hypouricemic agents), and electrolyte management before and following chemotherapy.

Hydration and Diuretics

The first and most important intervention to prevent TLS is hydration. Adequate hydration increases intravascular volume and improves renal blood flow and glomerular filtration rate. Thereafter, hydration decreases extracellular concentrations of uric acid, phosphorus, and potassium. Intravenous hydration should be started at least 24–48 h before chemotherapy initiation and continued during chemotherapy, depending on patient's clinical condition. In dangerous fluid overload cases, diuretics may be used to achieve urine output [82].

During pregnancy, hydration showed to be a possible and safe handling. However, a study showed that in some cases intravenous hydration significantly increased the amniotic fluid index of mothers with term pregnancy [83]. Since it caused no complications for the mother and fetus and with continuous monitoring of fluid balance, it can be used as an effective method in the management of TLS. Diuretics seems to be a safe management during pregnancy as well; a meta-analysis study of neonates exposed to diuretics during pregnancy did not find an increased risk of adverse effects, such as birth defects, fetal growth restriction, thrombocytopenia or diabetes [84]. Two types of diuretic agents are mainly used in obstetric practice: thiazide derivatives such as hydrochlorothiazide that act in inhibiting sodium and chloride reabsorption in distal renal tubules and collecting system. The other type of diuretic is furosemide with the advantage of a systemic as well as oral form of administration [85]. Diuretics may contribute to uric acid or calcium phosphate precipitation in renal tubules; hence, the patient must be well hydrated [80].

Hypouricemia Correction

Pharmacologic treatment of hypouricemia includes agents that decrease uric acid concentration in blood such as allopurinol, rasburicase, and febuxostat. Hypouricemic agents should be offered before, during, and after chemotherapy to avoid hypouricemia [80].

Allopurinol is a competitive inhibitor of xanthine oxidase, an enzyme responsible for the conversion of hypoxanthine to xanthine and of xanthine to uric acid. Although allopurinol is an effective inhibiting uric acid formation, it does not reduce existing uric acid level and may result in a build-up of xanthine and hypoxanthine concentration, leading to xanthine neuropathy [86]. Allopurinol use is related to some important chemotherapeutic drug interactions such as delayed catabolism of 6-mercaptopurin and azathioprine, in which dose should be reduced to one-third or one-fourth during allopurinol administration. In addition, it may also increase bone marrow toxicity after cyclophosphamide administration and reduced clearance of high methotrexate doses [87, 88]. Allopurinol use during pregnancy is still debated because there is not much evidence proving the safety and teratogenicity in fetus [89]. Therefore, some reported cases showed the safety of allopurinol use for TLS in pregnant women without complications related [90, 91].

Rasburicase or recombinant urate oxidase is a purified recombinant enzyme responsible for the breakdown of uric acid into allantoin, which is easily soluble and readily removed from blood. Rasburicase has a potentially reduced risk of contaminant-related allergic reaction, and action is faster when compared to allopurinol. The clinical use of rasburicase usually is limited due to its high cost and used in patients presenting with greatest risk of TLS or intolerant to allopurinol [92].

There are no data available about the use of rasburicase during pregnancy, but one case study showed the use of rasburicase in a pregnant woman (35 weeks) with no evidence of complications related to the delivery [93]. Rasburicase is contraindicated in patients with glucose-6-phosphate dehydrogenase (G6PD), a deficiency whose erythrocytes respond poorly to oxidative stress. Therefore, formal testing for G6PD deficiency is recommended before initiating rasburicase in patients [94, 95].

Febuxostat is a non-purine selective xanthine oxidase inhibitor approved for management of hyperuricemia. Febuxostat acts as a urate-lowering drug by inhibiting the production of urate from its purine precursors. It is a promising alternative to allopurinol in patients who are unable to tolerate allopurinol and decreases uric acid levels more effectively than allopurinol [96, 97]. There is a lack of studies about febuxostat use during pregnancy. It is classified in Pregnancy Category C and should be used during pregnancy only if the anticipated benefit justifies the risk to the fetus [98, 99].

Electrolytes Correction

Electrolyte management is related to the correction of hyperphosphatemia, hyperkalemia, and hypocalcemia. Electrolyte supplementation should be discontinued, especially those that include potassium and phosphorus should be stopped and removed from IV fluids [80]. Treatment of hyperphosphatemia includes intense hydration regimen and oral administration of phosphate binders as aluminum hydroxide, which will decrease the gut absorption of phosphate. The management of hyperphosphatemia will correct calcium levels, without the need for calcium infusion, avoiding the risk of precipitations of metastatic calcifications [100]. Aluminum administration during pregnancy can produce a syndrome that includes growth retardation, delayed ossification, and perhaps malformations at high doses. However, when given to mice and rabbits during organogenesis by gavage, aluminum hydroxide did not cause maternal or fetal toxic effects. A short use of aluminum compounds (8 weeks) is recommended [88, 101].

Treatment for hyperkalemia includes ECG monitoring and administration of sodium polystyrene sulfonate (SPS), hypertonic glucose and insulin, loop diuretics, and bicarbonate. Hyperkalemia can lead to potentially fatal cardiac dysrhythmias, and it is associated with increased mortality that necessitates cardiac monitoring. Loop diuretics can treat hyperkalemia by inhibiting potassium reabsorption at the loop of Henle. Insulin shifts potassium ions intracellularly, and glucose should be administered concomitantly to prevent hypoglycemia. Sodium bicarbonate shifts potassium intracellularly and slightly alkalinizes distal tubule secretion favoring the secretion, but it cannot be used during pregnancy due to clear risk of adverse events such as alkalosis [102]. During hyperphosphatemia, hypocalcemia should not be managed because of the increased risk of calcium-phosphate precipitation; if hypocalcemia is associated to symptoms, the clinician can decide on the necessity of calcium gluconate infusion [79, 103]. Sodium polystyrene sulfonate (SPS) is a cation exchange resin frequently used alone or in conjunction with the other therapies to lower serum potassium. SPS can be associated with bowel necrosis [104]. There are no studies in pregnant women using SPS, and it is classified as FDA Pregnancy Category C.

Dialysis

Patients who do not respond to the therapies already mentioned or experienced an acute renal failure will need renal replacement therapy such as hemodialysis. Dialysis manages electrolyte abnormalities, hyperuricemia, and treats renal failure associated to TLS. Frequent dialysis is recommended, considering the highly proliferative nature of cancer cells and the continual release of solute into blood stream. The timing and dose of dialysis should be linked to the purine generation rate; usually, daily dialysis is recommended until the crisis passes [92, 105]. Hemodialysis is the gold standard for substitution of renal function in women with chronic or acute renal insufficiency during pregnancy. For performing hemodialysis in pregnant women, it is most useful to use equipment which allows management of high blood flows (250–400 mL/min) and of dialysis fluid (600–800 mL/min) to be performed 4–6 sessions per week. It is recommended that new, unrecycled dialyzers (filters) of high biocompatibility and function be used, and the lowest possible dose of anticoagulant (heparin). Uterine activity should be monitored since fetal loss in the second and third trimesters of pregnancy is common in patients during or after hemodialysis [106].

9.2.4 Infections

Cancer patients receiving chemotherapy with reduced white blood cells, defined as neutropenia, is a common situation and increases the risk for infections [107]. Leukemia treatment also increases the risk of susceptibility to infections, cytopenia, and autoimmune phenomena during the chemotherapy. Chlorambucil has been utilized for the treatment of CLL for a long time, and the most infections reported are bacterial, most commonly respiratory. Purine analogs, such as fludarabine, cladribine, and pentostatin, induce T-cell abnormalities, and additionally purine analogues induce neutropenia. Bendamustine, another agent that can cause prolonged depletion of CD4 and CD8 cells, increases the risk of opportunistic infections in CLL patients. Therapy with monoclonal antibody, such as rituximab, also posed an increased risk for viral infections, and it can be higher in combination with fludarabine. Alemtuzumab, another monoclonal antibody, is associated with severe neutropenia as well as severe defects in cellular immunity [108, 109].

The most common infections associated with these agents include bacterial (mycobacterium, nocardia, listeria), fungal (candida, aspergillus), *Pneumocystis* , *Cryptococcus*, and viral, with cytomegalovirus (CMV), varicella zoster virus (VZV), and herpes simplex virus (HSV).

During pregnancy, the immune system changes, and this fact makes women more susceptible to infection. These episodes constitute a serious maternal and fetal risk, and not all antibiotics can be safely administered during pregnancy [3]. Pregnant women with leukemia, particularly acute leukemia (AL), present with anemia, thrombocytopenia, and neutropenia, in addition to recurrent infections due to bone marrow failure caused by the aggressive malignancy [5]. Potential risks from treatment of AL during pregnancy include, among other consequences, secondary infection, thrombocytopenia, and neutropenia. These maternal and fetal risks of both deferring therapy and proceeding with chemotherapy must be discussed with the patient, and all options including termination of the pregnancy must be weighed by the mother and a multidisciplinary healthcare team, including hematologists, obstetricians, and pediatricians [110, 111]. Induction with cytarabine and anthracycline in acute myeloid leukemia is associated with considerable maternal toxicity, including mucositis and prolonged neutropenia accompanied by bacterial and sometimes invasive fungal infections that require systemic therapy. Penicillin, cephalosporins, and metronidazole seem to be safe during pregnancy. Amphotericin B is the antifungal drug with the widest experience during pregnancy, with no reports of teratogenicity [112]. Voriconazole might be teratogenic as well, and evidence regarding the use of caspofungin and posaconazole is lacking [112]. Based on the available data, it seems that if treated with appropriate regimens, pregnant women with AML have outcomes like those of non-pregnant woman [113].

According to the National Comprehensive Cancer Network (NCCN) Guidelines for Clinical Practice in Oncology, it is recommended to do antimicrobial prophylaxis, based on overall infection risk in patients with cancer. Considering the intermediate risk in chronic lymphocytic leukemia (CLL) and the high risk for AL (induction and consolidation phase), the recommendation is bacterial, fungal, and viral prophylaxis [114]. There is insufficient evidence to support the use of routine antibiotics or antifungal and antiviral drugs during pregnancy to avoid the adverse effects of infections on pregnancy outcomes. Thus, treatment should be evaluated and decided with a focus on benefit against risk during symptoms.

Antifungal Treatment

Antifungal drugs are given as a routine preventive measure or when people who are at risk have a fever. Intravenous amphotericin B could reduce the number of deaths. Three of the drugs, amphotericin B, fluconazole, and itraconazole, reduced fungal infections. For antifungal treatment in patients with ALL, the NCCN has recommended fluconazole, micafungin, or amphotericin B. The same drugs or other option like posaconazole or voriconazole, after the observations of the risk and until the resolutions of neutropenia during AML treatment [114].

Azoles

The azoles drugs, such as fluconazole, voriconazole, and posaconazole, act by targeting the C14α demethylase and inhibiting the biosynthesis of ergosterol, an essential component of fungal cell membranes. Animal and human data provide evidence that these antifungal drugs could be teratogenic. Fluconazole, for example, can cross the placenta and is shown to be embryotoxic in rabbits, and embryo-fetotoxic and teratogenic in rats [115]. In this group, the classification of prescription drugs by the US FDA according to the risk in pregnancy is C for posaconazole, and D for voriconazole and fluconazole [112, 115, 116]. Yet, when the adverse symptoms include superficial fugus infections, the use of topical azoles, including bifonazole, clotrimazole, fenticonazole, isoconazole, ketoconazole, omoconazole, oxiconazole, sertaconazole, tioconazole, miconazole, and econazole, is allowed at any stage of pregnancy because they are not or are minimally absorbed [115].

Echinocandin

Micafungin, anidulafungin, and caspofungin are semi-synthetic cyclic hexapeptides that inhibit the 1,3-b-D-glucan synthase involved in fungal wall synthesis. These agents are available for intravenous administration only and are active against *Candida* spp. and *Aspergillus* spp. These drugs have best indication for treatment of severe infections, for patients who require hospitalization. The risk in pregnancy is C according to the FDA, with no human data; only animal studies have shown to be embryotoxic, and it is teratogenic in rabbits [112, 115, 117].

Polyenes

Classified as Category B by the FDA, the amphotericin B binds to ergosterol, forming transmembrane pores, leading to ionic leakage and finally to fungal death [112]. According to the NCCN recommendation, the lipid formulation is preferred based on less toxicity [114]. Case reports suggest that liposomal amphotericin B should also be considered as safe in pregnancy. Mueller et al. retrospectively evaluated liposomal amphotericin B and observed that its use in the first or second trimester in 16 patients caused no abortion, and no fetal malformations were reported [115, 118]. Despite these recommendations, there are no data with suggestions for the treatment of pregnant patients with leukemia who have developed fungal infections. Further studies with this specific type of population are needed.

Antiviral Treatment

Antiviral treatment is especially important to evaluate the presence of cytomegalovirus and herpes virus because of the increased risk of reactivation during leukemia and the potentially catastrophic neonatal complications [3]. The intermediate and high risks involving viral infection during leukemia require treatment. According to the NCCN recommendations, there is possible herpes simplex virus (HSV), varicella zoster virus (VZV), cytomegalovirus (CMV), hepatitis B and C (HBV and HCV), and human immunodeficiency virus (HIV) reaction or disease, during treatment with chemotherapy or targeted treatment like imatinib, nilotinib or ponatinib for CLL or ALL [114]. Furthermore, human influenza virus A and B can cause disease with a possibility of causing pneumonia, a secondary bacterial infection [119].

Herpes simplex virus is one of the most encountered viral infections in pregnancy and can cause maternal, fetal and neonatal infection. Nucleoside antiviral agents, including acyclovir, valacyclovir, famciclovir, ganciclovir, cidofovir, and ribavirin, are commonly used for the treatment, but acyclovir and valacyclovir are the drugs of choice for treatment of HSV infections during pregnancy. Both drugs are classified as Category B by the FDA [112, 120]. Acyclovir, considered as the drug of choice during pregnancy [121], is a nucleoside viral deoxyribonucleic acid

(DNA) polymerase inhibitor that is phosphorylated by viral thymidine kinase to the active triphosphate derivative and compete with deoxyguanosine triphosphate for incorporation into the viral DNA. Valacyclovir is the oral prodrug of acyclovir and is rapidly converted in vivo to acyclovir [112]. Cytomegalovirus, another member of the Herpesviridae Family, remains latent and can reactivate during chemotherapy. The treatment for non-pregnant patients includes ganciclovir or valganciclovir, cidofovir, and foscarnet, all of them classified as Category C by the FDA, and letermovir, not assigned by the US FDA pregnancy category, has not been recommended during pregnancy [112, 114]. Currently, there are no approved treatments for CMV in a pregnant woman [112, 120].

Although controversies still exist regarding reactivation of viral hepatitis in cancer patients, including HBV and HCV infections, prophylactic therapy is still recommended for this population according to clinical practice guidelines [114, 122, 123]. Among non-pregnant adults, first-line treatment for HBV is with the nucleoside or nucleotide analogue antivirals. Among pregnant women, HBV immunoglobulin, tenofovir, lamivudine, and telbivudine have been investigated as treatments to decrease the rate of congenital infection or maternal-to-child transmission. Studies of tenofovir, classified as Category B by the FDA, for the treatment of HBV during pregnancy have also reported positive effects, although there are fewer data than for lamivudine, classified as Category C by the FDA [120, 124]. Despite HCV, in general, women with HCV infection tolerate pregnancy well, and there are no recommendations for the treatment of active HCV in pregnancy [120].

Influenza is an acute respiratory illness caused by infection with influenza viruses. Human influenza A and B viruses cause mild respiratory illness with symptoms such as fever, myalgia (muscle pain), headache, cough, chills, nasal congestion, and sore throat. The major complication caused by influenza is pneumonia (secondary bacterial infection), and people with hematological cancers undergoing chemotherapy are at increased risk for influenza-related complications, in which hospitalizations are four times higher and mortality ten times higher among people with cancer when compared to the general population [119]. Pregnant women are also at high risk of developing influenza diseases. Despite that, oseltamivir and zanamivir act against influenza viruses A and B, and are commonly recommended for the treatment and chemoprophylaxis for influenza during pregnancy, although both drugs are classified as Category C by the FDA. Its action mechanism inhibits neuraminidase enzyme to prevent it from cleaving host-cell receptors and releasing newly synthesized virus [112].

Antibacterial Treatment
Bacteremic infections are the most common complications in patients with leukemia [125]. Despite pregnancy being associated with an increased susceptibility to infections, this risk is increased in patients with deficient hematological tumor and with chemotherapy treatment [111]. There was a reported case of a pregnant woman diagnosed with CLL, having recurrent respiratory tract infection episodes [126]. Patients with acute leukemia clinically present with frequent fever and respiratory

infections before chemotherapy, and virtually all patients develop problems, with infection and hemorrhage after treatment of leukemia. The empiric regimens include antipseudomonal penicillins and aminoglycosides, or more recently monotherapy with a third-generation cephalosporin such as ceftazidime can be used [127]. But the treatment of infection in pregnant women should consider the risks and benefits for the mother and the fetus.

The class of penicillin drugs freely crosses the placenta with no harmful fetal effects [127], but the combination with clavulanate is frequently used in cancer patients. It is better to avoid it to prevent problems for the newborn. In case of allergy to penicillin, clarithromycin can be used as an alternative. Cephalosporins and metronidazole could be safely used during pregnancy. On the other hand, aminoglycosides, quinolones, trimethoprim, and tetracyclines should be avoided [111, 113].

Penicillins

Penicillin is the most prescribed class of antimicrobials during pregnancy [128]. Penicillin inhibits enzymes that catalyze the final step in bacterial cell wall assembly, which forms the cross-links that bridge peptidoglycan, inhibiting bacterial cell wall synthesis [129, 130]. They are used against gram-positive streptococcal, staphylococcal, enterococcal, and meningococcal strains and are used in the treatment of syphilis, gonorrhea, and meningitis [129]. This class includes aminopenicillin, antipseudomonal penicillins, beta-lactamase inhibitors, natural penicillin, and penicillinase-resistant penicillin. According to the NCCN recommendations, piperacillin/tazobactam are the penicillin drugs used for treatment of bacterial infections in nonpregnancy cancer patients , with broad-spectrum activity against most gram-positive, gram-negative, and anaerobic organisms, and oral antibiotic combinations of amoxicillin/clavulanate, with spectrum against aerobic gram-positive organism and anaerobes, in combination with ciprofloxacin (see later) [114]. Both penicillins are classified as Category B in terms of risk during pregnancy by the FDA [131].

Cephalosporin

Cephalosporin is an alternative to penicillin for patients allergic or intolerant to penicillins, and it has a long history of documented use in pregnancy [128]. They are b-lactam antibiotics that inhibit bacterial cell wall synthesis and are commonly used in pregnancy, with a similar safety record to the penicillins. Cephalosporins belong to FDA Category B and are used to treat various infections such as urinary tract infection (UTI), pneumonia, otitis and sinusitis, and serious bacterial infections [129]. According to the NCCN guidelines, cefepime or ceftazidime is indicated. The first one with spectrum against most gram-positive and gram-negative organisms, and the second one with poor gram-positive activity, and both not active with most anaerobes and *Enterococcus* spp. [114].

If it is necessary to treat infections resulting from neutropenia related to leukemia or induced by chemotherapy, it is possible to consider the use of cephalosporins during pregnancy as well as the use of penicillin safe [128, 129].

Aminoglycosides

Aminoglycosides are highly efficacious drugs, particularly against gram-negative bacteria. The actions of aminoglycosides on bacteria are a multistep process, beginning at the plasma membrane, followed by an internalization and by effects on various intracellular processes. They bind to the 30s ribosomal sub-unit and can cause a misreading of the genetic code. This subsequently leads to the interruption of normal bacterial protein synthesis. Their original and major indications are against *Mycobacterium tuberculosis* and *Pseudomonas organism* [132].

According to the NCCN recommendations, the treatment with aminoglycosides, such as amikacin, gentamicin, or tobramycin, present spectrum activity primally against gram-negative organism [114]. Although this recommendation is for non-pregnant cancer patients, in case of pregnant women, aminoglycosides are FDA Pregnancy Category D, because of their potential nephro- and neurotoxicity to the fetus, and are acceptable only in cases when the expected benefits for the mother outweigh the risks to the unborn child [131]. In addition, the combination of aminoglycosides and cephalosporins should be avoided because there are proven studies suggesting nephrotoxicity [129].

Quinolone

Quinolones are another class of antibiotics that can be used during cancer therapy in non-pregnant patients [114]. Quinolones act by converting their targets, gyrase, and topoisomerase IV, into toxic enzymes that fragment the bacterial chromosome [133]. Ciprofloxacin (associated with amoxicillin/clavulanate), levofloxacin, and moxifloxacin are quinolone drugs that are active against gram-negative and atypical organisms [114]. Quinolones are a group of synthetic antibacterial agents classed as Category C by the FDA. There is a suggested association with quinolones and renal toxicity, cardiac defects, and central nervous system toxicity in the fetus [129, 134]. Muanda and colleagues demonstrated that quinolones and other antibiotics, such as macrolides (excluding erythromycin), tetracyclines, sulfonamides, and metronidazole, during early pregnancy were associated with an increased risk of spontaneous abortion [128]. In contrast, a number of studies have demonstrated exposure to quinolones during the first trimester to be safe. Overall, with uncertain evidence, the use of quinolones in pregnancy is only recommended if there is no alternative, and termination of pregnancy following exposure is not indicated [129, 134].

Others Antibacterial Agents

Other antibacterial agents, such as vancomycin, daptomycin, linezolid, imipenem/cilastatin, meropenem, metronidazole, and trimethoprim/sulfamethoxazole, are present in the guidelines, indicating the treatment of infections during chemotherapy of non-pregnant patients [114].

Vancomycin, a glycopeptide agent, inhibits the synthesis of peptidoglycans involved in stabilizing the bacterial cell wall [135]. Active spectrum against gram-positive organisms [114] is classed as Category B by the FDA, and it can cross placental barrier [131, 135] but appears to be safe and effective in the case of serious gram-positive infections, particularly during the second and third trimesters. There is limited information available about vancomycin use in the first trimester; caution is warranted during this period [134].

Carbapenem drugs, including ertapenem, meropenem, and doripenem, are Pregnancy Category B, while imipenem-cilastatin is Pregnancy Category C, by the FDA. According NCCN recommendations for non-pregnant cancer patients, the broad-spectrum activity is against most gram-positive, gram-negative, and anaerobic organisms [114]. The use in therapy should be reserved for pregnant women with infections that are resistant to penicillin and cephalosporin therapy with limited alternatives [131, 134].

Linezolid, an oxazolidinone, is Pregnancy Category C [131, 134] and suitable for targeted therapy of infections, caused by methicillin-resistant or glycopeptide gram-positive, and is also an alternative for the treatment of nocardiosis and listeriosis. It is also recommended against gram-positive organisms, including vancomycin-resistant enterococci[114]. Although some case reports are related to positive maternal outcomes without fetal teratogenesis of 4 weeks of linezolid use starting on second trimester of pregnancy [134], there are still insufficient data regarding administration during pregnancy. Hence, this antibiotic is not recommended during pregnancy or should be considered for use during pregnancy only when potential benefits outweigh the risks [134, 135].

Daptomycin is a cyclic lipopeptide, which is effective against gram-positive organisms, and is Pregnancy Category B [131, 134]. Isolated reports suggest that daptomycin may be safe to use on second and third trimesters [134]. However, there are still insufficient data regarding administration during pregnancy; it should be used in pregnancy only if the benefits outweigh the risks [134, 135].

Metronidazole is classified as Pregnancy Category B [134]. However, it is contraindicated, especially in the first trimester of pregnancy because its relationship with preterm birth, during early pregnancy, was associated with an increased risk of spontaneous abortion [128], and addition of few records with its association with childhood neuroblastoma [129, 134, 135]. Metronidazole inhibits DNA synthesis [135] and crosses the placenta barrier. It is used in the treatment of anaerobic (they associate with others antibacterial agents) and protozoal infections [129]. Despite some related risks, metronidazole also remains a recommended therapy for bacterial vaginosis and trichomonas infections in pregnancy [134].

Sulfamethoxazole and trimethoprim are both classed as Pregnancy Category C by the FDA. They can cross the placenta and should be avoided in the first trimester due to the mechanism of trimethoprim as a folate antagonist, and the exposure during this period can significantly increase the risk of congenital malformations (especially in neural tube) and cardiac defects. Regarding the third trimester of pregnancy, it should also be avoided due to the risk of an increase in unbound bilirubin due to competitive protein binding [134] and can cause kernicterus due to the displacement of bilirubin in the newborn if administered shortly before birth [135]. Overall, sulfamethoxazole-trimethoprim should be avoided in the first trimester and in the second and third trimesters, and should be used in pregnancy only if the benefits outweigh the risks and if other treatment options are available [134].

9.2.5 Neuropathy

Some cancer treatments can cause peripheral neuropathy (PN), a damage to nerves of the peripheral nervous system, which transmits information from the brain and spinal cord to every other part of the body. It is caused by morphologic or functional abnormalities in peripheral nerves and is separated into axonopathy (axonal abnormalities) or myelinopathy (myelin sheath abnormalities) [136].

The causes of peripheral neuropathy can include certain chemotherapeutic agents, such as vincristine, cytarabine, interferon, or methotrexate; systemic disease such as deficient vitamins, like thiamine, B12, pyridoxine, niacin, and vitamin E; and infectious or autoimmune diseases such as herpes zoster, herpes simplex, and cytomegalovirus [137].

Peripheral neuropathy is rare in pregnant patients, and the data about the neuropathy induced by chemotherapy in pregnant women during leukemia treatment are scarce.

Effective PN treatment is lacking, and therefore treatment options are limited. The antioxidant glutathione has been considered, but there is no significant improvement in measured outcomes when compared with results with placebo. In terms of PN pain, the selective serotonin-norepinephrine reuptake inhibitor duloxetine has shown promise. A double-blinded, placebo-controlled, crossover trial found that duloxetine 60 mg daily had a beneficial effect, and this was more recently confirmed in a study comparing duloxetine and vitamin B12 [138]. Treatment with vitamin E may reduce neurotoxicity, especially cisplatin-induced neurotoxicity. It was associated with significantly lower incidence of neuropathy compared with no supplementation [136].

9.2.6 Inflammatory Processes, Fever, and Pain

Patients with leukemia typically present with symptoms witnessed in chronic inflammatory diseases, such as fatigue, fever, night sweats, weight loss, bone pain, or abdominal pain, especially in acute leukemia and B-cell chronic lymphocytic leukemia (CLL) [127, 139]. These symptoms during pregnancy may represent the possibility of consequences for the offspring.

Adverse outcomes may be due to infections that culminate in fever. This fever during the first trimester has been linked to brain damage and neural tube defects; during the second trimester to autism spectrum disorder and lack of task persistence, besides associations between maternal fever and attention deficit hyperactivity disorder among offspring [139].

Regarding inflammatory processes, dysregulation of the immune system that produces an exaggerated inflammatory response, associated with an inadequate response to infectious stimuli, in addition to reinforcing the evolution of, mainly, chronic lymphocytic leukemia (CLL) [140]. Despite that, in pregnant women the inflammatory processes are implicated to early pregnancy (implantation and decidualization) to later during labor [141].

The association of pain and leukemia, especially acute leukemia, was investigated by Shaulov and colleagues. It was observed that pain occurs after beginning of induction chemotherapy, and the severe pain was associated with younger age, poorer performance status, a diagnosis of ALL, and time from onset of chemotherapy, with pain increasing sharply from 2 weeks to 4–5 weeks after initiation of chemotherapy [142].

There are few studies that validate oncologic pain during pregnancy, but the treatment of pain during pregnancy, as chronic, acute, or severe pain, is already well established with data on safe use of medications that can also be used to treat inflammatory processes and fever [143]. The available treatments involve steroidal and nonsteroidal anti-inflammatory drugs, and it should be used with care in pregnant patients.

Nonsteroidal Anti-inflammatory Drugs

Non-steroidal anti-inflammatory drugs (NSAIDs) are among the most widely used drugs in the developed world to treat pain, fever, and inflammatory processes and are often used by pregnant women [144].

The use of nonsteroidal anti-inflammatory drugs (NSAIDs), including drugs such as ibuprofen, naproxen, and ketorolac, during pregnancy, especially around conception, is associated with increased miscarriage risk, and the use in late pregnancy is generally avoided because it is associated with a substantial increase in the risk of premature ductal closure via their inhibition of prostaglandin E2 production [144–146]. The second trimester use of NSAIDs appears relatively safe, although the identification of an association with infant cryptorchidism, in addition, may be associated with neonatal renal impairment in premature infants, as the use on third-trimester NSAID. Many practitioners consider these drugs unsuitable for use after 28–32 weeks' gestation. The NSAIDs are rated Category B, by the FDA [147].

Paracetamol (acetaminophen) has demonstrated efficacy and apparent safety at all stages of pregnancy in standard therapeutic doses and is a first-line analgesic [145, 146]. The probable mechanism of effect to be safe is that paracetamol inhibits prostaglandin biosynthesis only in the central nervous system, whereas other NSAIDs inhibit prostaglandin biosynthesis in most organ systems [144].

Aspirin on high doses (> 1 g/day) decreased mean birth weight and fetal abnormalities, including cerebral hemorrhage, constricted ductus arteriosus, neonatal acidosis, and neonatal salicylate toxicity, whereas low-dose aspirin has been extensively used to prevent hypertension, pre-eclampsia, preterm birth, intrauterine growth restriction, and perinatal death [143]. But the relationship between aspirin and birth defects remains also controversial, and more investigations must be done. The low-dose aspirin is classed on Category C, but doses > 150 mg/day are Category D, by the FDA [147].

Indomethacin appears to be safe [146]. It has a potent inhibitory effect on uterine contractions and can reduce the risk of preterm birth during the second trimester [147].

Diclofenac is also used during early pregnancy if paracetamol or ibuprofen are not effective as analgesic to treat moderate pain. Diclofenac has analgesic, anti-inflammatory and antipyretic properties due to inhibition of cyclooxygenase-1 and cyclooxygenase-2, which leads to a reduced prostaglandin synthesis—as any other NSAIDs. It should be avoided in the third trimester due the increased risk of feto-toxic effects [148].

Dipyrone, taken out from the US market, is still available in some European and Latin American countries. In Brazil it is widely used, and there is no association found with major fetal malformations, intrauterine death, or preterm delivery. In contrast, in other studies, it has been associated with Wilms tumors in children exposed in utero, and there are several case reports, suggesting its association with oligohydramnios and closure of the ductus arteriosus when used in the third trimester, like other NSAIDs [149].

Corticoids

Corticosteroids are commonly prescribed in cancer patients for a variety of symptoms, including hypercalcemia and non-specific indications such as adjuvant analgesics in pain, management of nausea and vomiting, fatigue, cancer-induced anorexia-cachexia, depressed mood, or poor general well-being and dyspnea [150].

Steroids can reduce pain, especially from inflammatory processes, intensity by inhibiting prostaglandin synthesis and reducing vascular permeability. This inhibition of the expression enzyme involved in tissue degeneration during inflammatory processes reduces proinflammatory cytokines and blocks the production of eicosanoids. As a consequence, corticosteroids are considered to be the most effective strategy against inflammatory pain [150].

During pregnancy, corticosteroids are administered due to their immunosuppressive and anti-inflammatory effects. Three of the most commonly used corticosteroids in pregnancy are prednisolone, dexamethasone, and betamethasone [151], classed by FDA as Categories B, C, and C, respectively [121]. Betamethasone and dexamethasone can cross the human placenta from the mother to the fetus [151]. Regarding some adverse effects during pregnancy, the use of corticoids can induce a modest increase in the risk of cleft lip with or without palate, increased risk of preterm birth, low birth weight, or pre-eclampsia, with little evidence, and insufficient evidence to determine whether systemic corticosteroids could contribute to gestational diabetes mellitus [152].

Opioids

Opioids include morphine-like agonists (e.g., morphine, hydromorphone, hydrocodone, codeine, and oxycodone), meperidine-like agonists and synthetic opioid analogues, such as tramadol, are suitable for more severe pain. If used close to delivery, they can result in neonatal withdrawal effects [146].

The use of narcotic analgesics in human pregnancies are limited, and there are no prospective, comparative studies. However, these drugs have been used in therapeutic doses by pregnant women for many years and there are limited data of increased risk of major or minor malformations, such as congenital heart disease, spina bifida, and club foot, or neonatal respiratory depression, and the neonatal abstinence syndrome (NAS) [145, 153]. The general recommendation is that opioid usage should be avoided, especially during the third trimester [154], or minimized during pregnancy and should never be considered as a first-line option [147]. According to the FDA, most opioids are Category B or C for short-term use, but during chronic or high-dose use in pregnancy, they become Category D [147, 155].

Other Analgesic Therapies
Anticonvulsants such as pregabalin is frequently used in chronic neuropathic pain, but there are no human studies that can help determine its safety in pregnancy. In rats, it has been associated with low-weight fetuses and bone problems. Antidepressants, such as fluoxetine has not been associated with fetal malformations and, if well tolerated by the mother, its use could be less risky than discontinuation. Among selective serotonin reuptake inhibitors (SSRIs), some authors suggest that sertraline is the safest due to its low levels in blood and mother's milk. Although there is an absolute risk of malformations, it is low when compared to other SSIRs [149].

Acupuncture has proved to be useful in musculoskeletal pain during pregnancy [149, 156]. In general, the overall consensus is that acupuncture's benefits outweigh its risks, and they can be considered in interested patients when the availability of other safe treatment options is limited [156]. Acupuncture requires the hands of a specialist with a continual avoidance of uterine and cervical reference points, in order to not trigger labor. Acupuncture also appears to be useful in the management of tension headache [149].

Activity modifications, physical exercise, and a physiotherapy program can be recommended in order to prevent low back pain [156]. When pain is already present, there are reports of good results with relaxation exercises and education on sleeping positions. Aerobic exercises in water help improve pain because of reduced gravitational loads on maternal muscles [149].

9.2.7 Fatigue

Fatigue has been reported to be highly prevalent in population-based surveys and in studies of some specific cancers and treatments. Severe fatigue has been reported more frequently in patients with hematologic malignancies than in patients with solid tumor, and this means a predictor of poor survival in a study of patients with chronic lymphocytic leukemia [157].

Fatigue severity might be greater in older or female patients, or in patients with poor performance status. In addition to fatigue, patients often report other symptoms caused by their disease or treatment, such as pain, infection, gastrointestinal (GI) symptoms, sleep disturbances, and body weight loss. Despite hematologic malignancies, more patients with acute leukemia (around 61%) reported severe fatigue compared with chronic leukemia patients (around 47%) and required better methods of fatigue management [157].

The relationship between fatigue and pregnancy is naturally established. Fatigue during early pregnancy typically gets better around the start of the second trimester. Pregnancy fatigue often returns in the third trimester, though it varies from pregnancy to pregnancy. Chien assessed the prevalence of fatigue in pregnant women and noted that 94.6% reported some symptom of fatigue, demonstrating a significant value for pregnant women [158].

Now, if there is a scenario with both conditions, a pregnant patient with hematologic malignancies, the intervention needs to be carefully carried out, as the symptoms can induce a confusion and slow up the real diagnosis. There are few case reports that discovered the diagnosis of leukemia next to the period of labor, common during the second and third trimester, due to the non-specific nature of the symptoms early during pregnancy [159]. In general, the management indicated to pregnant patients is relaxation techniques to help alleviate excess fatigue [160].

According to the NCCN recommendations, cases must be well evaluated, monitored, documented and treated in all age groups, all stages of the disease, before, during or after treatment [161]. There are some non-pharmacological interventions for patients who need fatigue management.

One of nonpharmacologic intervention is physical activity [161]. Health benefits of physical activity during and immediately after pregnancy include possible prevention of gestational diabetes, pre-eclampsia, and chronic musculoskeletal conditions, support of healthy weight and improved mental health [162]. In addition to that, some studies suggest that exercise, as well as behavioral and some psychosocial interventions, may reduce fatigue and improve the performance status of cancer patients, despite hematological malignancies; this activity reduces the treatment-related loss of physical performance in patients undergoing chemotherapy [163].

Other nonpharmacologic interventions include massage therapy, physical intervention (such as cognitive behavioral therapy to reduce the negative thoughts and emotions about the disease), nutrition consultation, and cognitive behavioral therapy for sleep [161].

Regarding pharmacological treatment, psychostimulants (methylphenidate and modafinil) have been used, to reduce the fatigue in patients with chronic diseases and may eventually be useful in some cancer patients [161, 163]. Methylphenidate, a stimulant drug derived from the amphetamine family, is an effective first-line treatment for attention deficit and hyperactivity disorder (ADHD). Although there are a few studies during pregnancy, the available data suggest no increase in the risk of malformation when used at therapeutic doses; however, there is an increased risk of low birth weight or preterm birth [164]. Modafinil is a stimulant used for the treatment of narcolepsy, and due the pregnancy safety category for modafinil remained undefined, the decision to continue or withhold medications for narcolepsy should be made by an informed patient, weighing the risks and benefits outlined [165].

When fatigue has another recognized origin, such as anemia or infection, the correct and appropriate treatment must be performed in pregnant patients.

9.2.8 Anemia

Anemia is the most frequent hematologic disorder affecting pregnant women. According to World health organization (WHO), 40% of pregnant women worldwide are anemic. In this condition, the number of red blood cells or the hemoglobin level (and its oxygen-carrying capacity) is reduced when compared to normal levels [166]. Generally, anemia occurs as a consequence of nutrition deficiency or congenital hemoglobinopathies [167].

In leukemias, accumulation of defective cells on the bone marrow reduces the production of red blood cells causing anemia, leading to symptoms such as fatigue, weakness, dizziness, and shortness of breath. Anemia treatment depends on the type, cause, and severity of the condition. Treatments can include nutrient reposition with dietary changes, use of supplements like iron or vitamin B, blood and blood products, and hormonal therapies.

Minerals and Vitamins
Iron administration is the first-line treatment for iron-deficient anemia. There are several commercial oral iron salts supplements in two main administration routes: oral and intravenous. WHO recommends a daily oral dose from 30 mg to 60 mg of elemental iron and 0.4 mg of folic acid to prevent maternal anemia, puerperal sepsis, low birth weight, and preterm birth. When anemia is diagnosed during pregnancy, elemental iron daily dose should be 120 mg until hemoglobin level is $\geq$ 11 g/dL [166].

Iron's oral administration is limited, and its absorption is effective only when there are no problems with the intestinal uptake. Parenteral administration is the most effective route when faster depletion and quicker response are desired and when oral supplementation is ineffective [168]. In most of the cases, iron is considered safe for use in pregnant women and is constantly used as a component of prenatal vitamin and mineral supplements. Iron absorption increases with a diet rich in ascorbic acid, red meat, and fish and reduces when the diet is rich in calcium and polyphenols [167].

Treatment of anemia caused by folate deficiency and/or vitamin B12 (including megaloblastic anemias) generally responds to treatment with folic acid and/or hydroxocobalamin/ cyanocobalamin [169].

Folate deficiency caused by drugs that inhibit dihydrofolate reductase (e.g., methotrexate) needs to "bypass" this enzyme blockade, giving the synthetic folinic acid. Folinic acid rescue therapy reduces toxic effects on healthy tissues of high-dose methotrexate used in cancer treatment. Folinic acid is given orally, usually as calcium folinate salt [169].

Transfusion
Red cell transfusion is almost always required to replace hemoglobin levels when they are less than 6 g/dL in obstetric hemorrhages, antenatal and postnatal anemia [170].

Risks involving transfusion are circulatory overload, transfusion reactions, incompatibility, and infections. Electrolyte imbalance can also occur as a result of blood transfusions, especially hyperkalemia and hypocalcemia. The decision of transfusion must consider patient's consent, clinical history, and hemoglobin level (levels less than 5 g/dL implies high risk of mortality) [171]. It is important to receive a blood transfusion before severe anemia develops [170].

Transfusion-Related Iron Excess Treatment

In transfusion-dependent patients, like in cases of myelodysplastic syndrome and β-thalassemia, iron overload can be a clinical concern. Chelation therapy is an efficient way to deplete iron excess. Iron chelators currently used in clinical practice are deferoxamine, deferiprone, and deferasirox, but their use during gestation is contraindicated and information about safe usage during pregnancy is scarce [172]. Despite some cases of inadvertently pregnant exposure to chelators during a short period of gestation did not prevent the arrival of healthy babies, their use in pregnancy should be considered only when potential benefits outweigh potential risks to the fetus [173].

Granulocyte Stimulators

Granulocyte colony-stimulating factor (G-CSF) is a type of growth factor used to recover the number of white blood cells (mainly neutrophils), like in chemotherapy treatment, stem cell transplant, and aplastic anemia.

There are several types of therapeutic G-CSF produced by recombinant DNA technology:

- Filgrastim (recombinant human G-CSF)
- Lenograstim (glycosylated recombinant G-CSF)
- Pegfilgrastim and lipegfilgrastim (long-acting pegylated forms)

G-CSFs are administered by subcutaneous injection or intravenous infusion. Usually, lenograstim and filgrastim are given daily until the neutrophil numbers recover, and pegylated forms are given once after chemotherapy [169].

Although studies suggest filgrastim may cross the placental barrier, there is no strong evidence of congenital toxicity related to the use of G-CSF in humans, and also they were not teratogenic in rats [174].

Adverse effects of G-CSF are falcemic crisis (acute and painful) in patients with falciforme anemia, nausea, vomiting, headache, and bone pain.

Erythropoietin

Erythropoietin is a hormone that stimulates formation and release of red blood cells from the bone marrow, resulting in the rise of hematocrit. Therapeutic erythropoietin is produced using DNA recombinant technology and is also found in a hyperglicosylated form darbaphoetin alpha and methoxy polyethylene glycol-epoetin beta, which have longer half-life [169].

Erythropoietin is used in treatment of anemia, including anemia in chronic kidney disease, myelodysplasia, and cancer chemotherapy. Minimum adverse effects were observed in using erythropoietin combined with iron to treat iron-deficiency anemia in pregnancy [175, 176].

Erythropoietin has some advantages over blood transfusion treatment [177]:

- No risk of transfusion reaction
- More acceptability to patients (including the ones with religious objections, e.g., Jehovah's Witnesses)
- Reduced risks of infections
- Decreased consumption of blood products
- Decrease in the necessity for hospitalization

9.2.9   Gastrointestinal Problems

Gastrointestinal problems like nauseas and vomiting, hyperemesis gravidarum, gastroesophageal reflux disease, constipation, and diarrhea are common during pregnancy [178].

In gastroesophageal reflux disease (GERD), the gastric content passes through the esophagus, causing damage to the mucosa and symptoms like heartburn [179]. GERD can be intrinsic related to pregnancy because it causes modification of visceral anatomy, affecting normal motility of esophagus, stomach, and intestines, or it is related to chronic gastrointestinal disorders [180].

Lifestyle and dietary modifications such as avoiding smoking, drinking alcohol, eating spicy and fatty foods, chocolate, caffeine, and mints may not be enough in GERD treatment, and medicines like antacids, H2 inhibitors and proton pump inhibitors may be necessary [180].

Antacids
Antacids are preferred by patients because it provides fast symptomatic relief and can be used on demand. Aluminum, magnesium, and calcium antacids are commonly used for treating GERD and are considered safe during pregnancy at usual doses [181]. No teratogenic effects of these drugs have been observed in animal studies [182]. Bicarbonate-containing antacids should be avoided because it can precipitate metabolic alkalosis and fluid overload in the mother and fetus [183]. Calcium-based antacids are recommended in pregnancy because of its safe record, and it can increase calcium intake, which has been associated with prevention of pre-eclampsia [184].

Histamine-2 Receptor Antagonists
Histamine-2 receptor antagonists (H2RAs) are used to treat reflux symptoms not responding to antacids. Ranitidine, cimetidine, nizatidine, and famotidine are FDA-approved Category B for use in pregnancy. Cimetidine and ranitidine have been used in pregnancy for more than 30 years, presenting great safety profiles, but only ranitidine has efficacy proved during pregnancy.

No reports of sexual abnormalities in infants after exposure to cimetidine or other H2RAs were related, although past studies with cimetidine presented weak antiandrogenic effect in animals and was associated with gynecomastia in adult men [178].

Proton Pump Inhibitors

Proton pump inhibitors (PPIs), for example, omeprazole, lansoprazole, and pantoprazole, interact with H-K-ATPase and are one of the most effective therapies to control gastric acid secretion.

Despite early studies with omeprazole presenting dose-related embryonic and fetal toxicity in animals, recent studies in humans did not associate risk of major birth defects to any specific PPI. Currently, use of all PPIs in pregnancy is considered safe, and they are generally reserved for GERD complications or in not-responding treatments with antacids and H2RAs. Considering that iron absorption can be reduced with the usage of agents that decrease gastric acidity, PPIs should be used with caution [181].

References

1. Pecatorri FA, et al. ESMO Clinical Practice Guidelines for diagnosis, treatment and follow-up. Ann Oncol. 2013;24(Supplement 6):vi160–70. https://doi.org/10.1093/annonc/mdt199.
2. Saleh AJM, et al. Leukemia during pregnancy: long term follow up of 32 cases from a single institution. Hematol Oncol Stem Cell Ther. 2014;7(2):63–8.
3. Cuan-Baltazar Y, et al. Leukemia during pregnancy. Obstet Gynecol Int J. 2017;6(6):00225.
4. Fey MF, Surbeck D. Leukaemia and pregnancy. In: Surbone A, et al., editors. Cancer and pregnancy. New York: Springer Berlin Heidelberg; 2008.
5. Al-Anazi KA. Update on leukemia in pregnancy. In: Guenova M, editor. Leukemias – updates and new insights. London: IntechOpen; 2015.
6. Giagounidis AAN. Acute promyelocytic leukemia and pregnancy. Eur J Haematol. 2000;64:267–71.
7. FDA. Content and format of labeling for human prescription drug and biological products; Requirements for pregnancy and lactation labeling. Final rule. Fed Regist. 2014;79(233):72063–103.
8. Paydas S. Management of hemopoietic neoplasias during pregnancy. Crit Rev Oncol Hematol. 2016; https://doi.org/10.1016/j.critrevonc.2016.05.006.
9. Brenner B, Avivi I, Lishner M. Haematological cancers in pregnancy. Lancet. 2012; https://doi.org/10.1016/S0140-6736(11)61348-2.
10. Einarson A, et al. The safety of ondansetron for nausea and vomiting of pregnancy: a prospective comparative study. BJOG. 2004; https://doi.org/10.1111/j.1471-0528.2004.00236.x.
11. Shankar A, et al. Prevention of chemotherapy-induced nausea and vomiting in cancer patients. Asian Pac J Cancer Prev. 2015;16(15):6207–13.
12. Herrstedt J. The latest consensus on antiemetics. Curr Opin Oncol. 2018; https://doi.org/10.1097/CCO.0000000000000450.
13. Yokoe T, et al. Effectiveness of antiemetic regimens for highly emetogenic chemotherapy-induced nausea and vomiting: a systematic review and network meta-analysis. Oncologist. 2019; https://doi.org/10.1634/theoncologist.2018-0140.

14. Karthaus M, et al. Neurokinin-1 receptor antagonists: review of their role for the prevention of chemotherapy-induced nausea and vomiting in adults. Expert Rev Clin Pharmacol. 2019;12(7):661–80. https://doi.org/10.1080/17512433.2019.1621162. Available in: https://www.tandfonline.com/doi/full/10.1080/17512433.2019.1621162.
15. Singh P, Yoon SS, Kuo B. Nausea: a review of pathophysiology and therapeutics. Ther Adv Gastroenterol. 2016; https://doi.org/10.1177/1756283X15618131.
16. Theriot J, Wermuth HR, Ashurst JV. Antiemetic serotonin-5-HT3 receptor blockers. Treasure Island: StatPearls Publishing; 2019.
17. Choi BS, et al. Multicenter phase IV study of palonosetron in the prevention of chemotherapy-induced nausea and vomiting (CINV) in patients with non-Hodgkin lymphomas undergoing repeated cycles of moderately emetogenic chemotherapy. Leuk Lymphoma. 2014;55(3):544–50.
18. Simino GPR, et al. Efficacy, safety and effectiveness of ondansetron compared to other serotonin-3 receptor antagonists (5-HT3RAs) used to control chemotherapy-induced nausea and vomiting: systematic review and meta-analysis. Expert Rev Clin Pharmacol. 2016; https://doi.org/10.1080/17512433.2016.1190271.
19. Siminerio LL, et al. Ondansetron use in pregnancy. Obstet Gynecol. 2016; https://doi.org/10.1097/AOG.0000000000001375.
20. Lavecchia M, et al. Ondansetron in pregnancy and the risk of congenital malformations: a systematic review. J Obstet Gynaecol Can. 2018; https://doi.org/10.1016/j.jogc.2017.10.024.
21. Caritis S, et al. Pharmacodynamics of transdermal granisetron in women with nausea and vomiting of pregnancy. Am J Obstet Gynecol. 2016; https://doi.org/10.1016/j.ajog.2016.01.163.
22. Shapira M, et al. The safety of early pregnancy exposure to granisetron. Eur J Obstet Gynecol Reprod Biol. 2020;245:35–8. https://doi.org/10.1016/j.ejogrb.2019.11.033. Available in: https://linkinghub.elsevier.com/retrieve/pii/S0301211519305482.
23. Navari RM. Palonosetron: a second-generation 5-hydroxytryptamine receptor antagonist. Future Oncol. 2006; https://doi.org/10.2217/14796694.2.5.591.
24. Raedle LA. Akynzeo (netupitant and palonosetron), a dual-acting oral agent, approved by the FDA for the prevention of chemotherapy-induced nausea and vomiting. Am Health Drug Benefits. 2015;8:44–8.
25. Roila F, et al. 2016 MASCC and ESMO guideline update for the prevention of chemotherapy- and radiotherapy-induced nausea and vomiting and of nausea and vomiting in advanced cancer patients. Ann Oncol. 2016; https://doi.org/10.1093/annonc/mdw270.
26. Welliver M. Dopamine antagonists for nausea and vomiting: special considerations. Gastroenterol Nurs. 2014;37(5):361–4. https://doi.org/10.1097/SGA.0000000000000068.
27. Berkovitch M, et al. Metoclopramide for nausea and vomiting of pregnancy: a prospective multicenter international study. Am J Perinatol. 2002; https://doi.org/10.1055/s-2002-34469.
28. Matok I, et al. The safety of metoclopramide use in the first trimester of pregnancy. N Engl J Med. 2009; https://doi.org/10.1056/NEJMoa0807154.
29. Matok I, Perlman A. Metoclopramide in pregnancy: no association with adverse fetal and neonatal outcomes. Evid Based Med. 2014;19(3):115. https://doi.org/10.1136/eb-2013-101654. Available in: http://ebm.bmj.com/lookup/doi/10.1136/eb-2013-101654.
30. Mcparlin C, et al. Treatments for hyperemesis gravidarum and nausea and vomiting in pregnancy: a systematic review. JAMA. 2016; https://doi.org/10.1001/jama.2016.14337.
31. Pasternak B, et al. Metoclopramide in pregnancy and risk of major congenital malformations and fetal death. JAMA. 2013; https://doi.org/10.1001/jama.2013.278343.
32. Kashifard M, et al. Ondansetrone or metoclopromide? Which is more effective in severe nausea and vomiting of pregnancy? A randomized trial double-blind study. Clin Exp Obstet Gynecol. 2013;40(1):127–30.
33. Lachi-Silva L, et al. Population pharmacokinetics of orally administrated bromopride: focus on the absorption process. Eur J Pharm Sci. 2020; https://doi.org/10.1016/j.ejps.2019.105081.
34. Epifanio M, et al. Bromopride, metoclopramide, or ondansetron for the treatment of vomiting in the pediatric emergency department: a randomized controlled trial. J Pediatr. 2018; https://doi.org/10.1016/j.jped.2017.06.004.

35. Araújo JR. Gestação, Avaliação do bromopride nas náuseas e vômitos da gestação. J Bras Ginecol. 1981;91(4):283–5.
36. Babaei AH, Foghaha MH. A randomized comparison of vitamin B6 and dimenhydrinate in the treatment of nausea and vomiting in early pregnancy. Iran J Nurs Midwifery Res. 2014;19(2):199–202. Available in: http://www.ncbi.nlm.nih.gov/pubmed/24834091.
37. Slaughter SR, et al. FDA approval of doxylamine-pyridoxine therapy for use in pregnancy. N Engl J Med. 2014; https://doi.org/10.1056/NEJMp1316042.
38. Koren G, et al. Effectiveness of delayed-release doxylamine and pyridoxine for nausea and vomiting of pregnancy: a randomized placebo controlled trial. Am J Obstet Gynecol. 2010; https://doi.org/10.1016/j.ajog.2010.07.030.
39. Sripramote M, Lekhyananda N. A randomized comparison of ginger and vitamin B6 in the treatment of nausea and vomiting of pregnancy. J Med Assoc Thail. 2003;86(9):846–53.
40. Pongrojpaw D, Somprasit C, Chanthasenanont A. A randomized comparison of ginger and dimenhydrinate in the treatment of nausea and vomiting in pregnancy. J Med Assoc Thail. 2007; https://doi.org/10.1016/j.ajog.2006.10.299.
41. Sharifzadeh F, et al. A comparison between the effects of ginger, pyridoxine (vitamin B6) and placebo for the treatment of the first trimester nausea and vomiting of pregnancy (NVP). J Matern Fetal Neonatal Med. 2018; https://doi.org/10.1080/14767058.2017.1344965.
42. Sripramote M, Lekhyananda N. A randomized comparison of ginger and vitamin B6 in the treatment of nausea and vomiting of pregnancy. J Med Assoc Thai. 2003;86(9):846–53.
43. Heitmann K, Nordeng H, Holst L. Safety of ginger use in pregnancy: results from a large population-based cohort study. Eur J Clin Pharmacol. 2013; https://doi.org/10.1007/s00228-012-1331-5.
44. Portnoi G, et al. Prospective comparative study of the safety and effectiveness of ginger for the treatment of nausea and vomiting in pregnancy. Am J Obstet Gynecol. 2003; https://doi.org/10.1067/S0002-9378(03)00649-5.
45. Choi JS, et al. Assessment of fetal and neonatal outcomes in the offspring of women who had been treated with dried ginger (Zingiberis rhizoma siccus) for a variety of illnesses during pregnancy. J Obstet Gynaecol. 2015; https://doi.org/10.3109/01443615.2014.941342.
46. Lindblad AJ, Koppula S. Ginger for nausea and vomiting of pregnancy. Can Fam Physician. 2016;62(2):145. Available in: http://www.ncbi.nlm.nih.gov/pubmed/26884528.
47. Mcmahon BJ, Kwaan HC. Thrombotic and bleeding complications associated with chemotherapy. Semin Thromb Hemost. 2012; https://doi.org/10.1055/s-0032-1328885.
48. Gifkins DM, et al. Incidence of major hemorrhage among CLL and mcl patients compared to the general elderly population: an analysis of the us SEER-medicare linked database. Blood. 2015;126(23):3268.
49. Franchini M, et al. Bleeding complications in patients with hematologic malignancies. Semin Thromb Hemost. 2013; https://doi.org/10.1055/s-0032-1331154.
50. Kekre N, Connors JM. Venous thromboembolism incidence in hematologic malignancies. Blood Rev. 2019; https://doi.org/10.1016/j.blre.2018.06.002.
51. Hunt BJ. The current place of tranexamic acid in the management of bleeding. Anaesthesia. 2015; https://doi.org/10.1111/anae.12910.
52. Olldashi F, et al. Effects of tranexamic acid on death, vascular occlusive events, and blood transfusion in trauma patients with significant haemorrhage (CRASH-2): a randomised, placebo-controlled trial. Lancet. 2010; https://doi.org/10.1016/S0140-6736(10)60835-5.
53. Ker K, Prieto-Merino D, Roberts I. Systematic review, meta-analysis and meta-regression of the effect of tranexamic acid on surgical blood loss. Br J Surg. 2013; https://doi.org/10.1002/bjs.9193.
54. Ker K, et al. Effect of tranexamic acid on surgical bleeding: systematic review and cumulative meta-analysis. BMJ. 2012; https://doi.org/10.1136/bmj.e3054.
55. Sentilhes L, et al. Tranexamic acid for the prevention of blood loss after vaginal delivery. N Engl J Med. 2018; https://doi.org/10.1056/NEJMoa1800942.
56. Xu J, Gao W, Ju Y. Tranexamic acid for the prevention of postpartum hemorrhage after cesarean section: a double-blind randomization trial. Arch Gynecol Obstet. 2013; https://doi.org/10.1007/s00404-012-2593-y.

57. Ducloy-Bouthors AS, et al. High-dose tranexamic acid reduces blood loss in postpartum haemorrhage. Crit Care. 2011; https://doi.org/10.1186/cc10143.
58. Peitsidis P, Kadir RA. Antifibrinolytic therapy with tranexamic acid in pregnancy and post-partum. Expert Opin Pharmacother. 2011; https://doi.org/10.1517/14656566.2011.545818.
59. Marchili MR, et al. Vitamin K deficiency: a case report and review of current guidelines. Ital J Pediatr. 2018; https://doi.org/10.1186/s13052-018-0474-0.
60. Shahrook S, et al. Vitamin K supplementation during pregnancy for improving out-comes: a systematic review and meta-analysis. Sci Rep. 2018; https://doi.org/10.1038/s41598-018-29616-y.
61. Shahrook S, et al. Vitamin K supplementation during pregnancy for improving outcomes. In: Mori R, editor. Cochrane database of systematic reviews. Chichester: Wiley; 2014. https://doi.org/10.1002/14651858.CD010920. Available in: http://doi.wiley.com/10.1002/14651858.CD010920.
62. Hill RM, Kennell JH, Barnes AC. Vitamin K administration and neonatal hyperbilirubine-mia of unknown etiology. A double-blind study. Am J Obstet Gynecol. 1961; https://doi.org/10.1016/0002-9378(61)90065-5.
63. Schwartz RN. Management of venous thromboembolism for patients with hematologic malignancies. J Adv Pract Oncol. 2017;8(3):297–302. Available in: http://www.ncbi.nlm.nih.gov/pubmed/29928555.
64. Many A, Koren G. Low-molecular-weight heparins during pregnancy. Can Fam Physician. 2005;51(2):199–201.
65. Jacobson B, et al. Safety and efficacy of enoxaparin in pregnancy: a systematic review and meta-analysis. Adv Ther. 2020; https://doi.org/10.1007/s12325-019-01124-z.
66. Annibali O, et al. Incidence of venous thromboembolism and use of anticoagulation in hematological malignancies: critical review of the literature. Crit Rev Oncol Hematol. 2018; https://doi.org/10.1016/j.critrevonc.2018.02.003.
67. Khanal N, et al. Use of low molecular weight heparin (LMWH) in thrombocyto-penic patients with hematologic malignancy-associated venous thromboembolism (VTE). Blood. 2015;126(23):3482. https://doi.org/10.1182/blood.V126.23.3482.3482. Available in: https://ashpublications.org/blood/article/126/23/3482/90793/Use-of-Low-Molecular-Weight-Heparin-LMWH-in.
68. Lu E, et al. The safety of low-molecular-weight heparin during and after pregnancy. Obstet Gynecol Surv. 2017; https://doi.org/10.1097/OGX.0000000000000505.
69. Shlomo M, et al. The fetal safety of enoxaparin use during pregnancy: a population-based retrospective cohort study. Drug Saf. 2017; https://doi.org/10.1007/s40264-017-0573-7.
70. Green D. Management of bleeding complications of hematologic malignancies. Semin Thromb Hemost. 2007; https://doi.org/10.1055/s-2007-976178.
71. Karanth L, et al. Desmopressin acetate (DDAVP) for preventing and treating acute bleeds during pregnancy in women with congenital bleeding disorders. Cochrane Database Syst Rev. 2019; https://doi.org/10.1002/14651858.CD009824.pub4.
72. Ray JG. DDAVP use during pregnancy: an analysis of its safety for mother and child. Obstet Gynecol Surv. 1998; https://doi.org/10.1097/00006254-199807000-00025.
73. Jansen AJG, et al. Postpartum hemorrhage and transfusion of blood and blood components. Obstet Gynecol Surv. 2005; https://doi.org/10.1097/01.ogx.0000180909.31293.cf.
74. Hull RD, et al. Long-term low-molecular-weight heparin versus usual care in proximal-vein thrombosis patients with cancer. Am J Med. 2006; https://doi.org/10.1016/j.amjmed.2006.02.022.
75. Verma D, et al. Vitamin K antagonism impairs the bone marrow microenvironment and hematopoiesis. Blood. 2019; https://doi.org/10.1182/blood.2018874214.
76. Abadi S, Einarson A, Koren G. Use of warfarin during pregnancy. Can Pharm J. 2002;48:695–7.
77. Walfisch A, Koren G. The "warfarin window" in pregnancy: the importance of half-life. J Obstet Gynaecol Can. 2010; https://doi.org/10.1016/S1701-2163(16)34689-8.
78. Marshall AL. Diagnosis, treatment, and prevention of venous thromboembolism in preg-nancy. Postgrad Med. 2014; https://doi.org/10.3810/pgm.2014.11.2830.

79. Criscuolo M, et al. Tumor lysis syndrome: review of pathogenesis, risk factors and management of a medical emergency. Expert Rev Hematol. 2016; https://doi.org/10.1586/1747408 6.2016.1127156.
80. Belay Y, Yirdaw K, Enawgaw B. Tumor lysis syndrome in patients with hematological malignancies. J Oncol. 2017; https://doi.org/10.1155/2017/9684909.
81. Cairo MS, Bishop M. Tumour lysis syndrome: new therapeutic strategies and classification. Br J Haematol. 2004; https://doi.org/10.1111/j.1365-2141.2004.05094.x.
82. Coiffier B, et al. Guidelines for the management of pediatric and adult tumor lysis syndrome: an evidence-based review. J Clin Oncol. 2008; https://doi.org/10.1200/JCO.2007.15.0177.
83. Shahnazi M, et al. The effects of intravenous hydration on amniotic fluid volume and pregnancy outcomes in women with term pregnancy and oligohydramnios: a randomized clinical trial. J Caring Sci. 2012; https://doi.org/10.5681/jcs.2012.018.
84. Al-Balas M, Bozzo P, Einarson A. Use of diuretics during pregnancy. Can Fam Physician. 2009;55(1):44–5.
85. Barrilleaux PS, Martin JN. Hypertension therapy during pregnancy. Clin Obstet Gynecol. 2002;45(1):22–34. https://doi.org/10.1097/00003081-200203000-00005. Available in: http://journals.lww.com/00003081-200203000-00005.
86. Larosa C, et al. Acute renal failure from xanthine nephropathy during management of acute leukemia. Pediatr Nephrol. 2007; https://doi.org/10.1007/s00467-006-0287-z.
87. Alhubaishi AA. Pancytopenia and septic infection caused by concurrent use of allopurinol and mercaptopurine: a case report illustrating the importance of clinical pharmacist consultation. Am J Case Rep. 2019; https://doi.org/10.12659/AJCR.914166.
88. Sánchez Gómez E, Arco Prados Y. Review of pharmacological interactions of oral anticancer drugs provided at pharmacy department. Farm Hosp. 2014; https://doi.org/10.7399/fh.2014.38.4.1157.
89. Simsek M, et al. The teratogenicity of allopurinol: a comprehensive review of animal and human studies. Reprod Toxicol. 2018; https://doi.org/10.1016/j.reprotox.2018.08.012.
90. Álvarez-Goris MDP, et al. Síndrome de lisis tumoral en un embarazo complicado con leucemia linfoblástica aguda. Ginecol Obstet Mex. 2016;84(4):252–6.
91. El-Sonbaty MR, Bitar Z, Abdulrazak A. Acute spontaneous tumor-lysis syndrome in a pregnant woman with non-Hodgkin's lymphoma. Int J Hematol. 2001;73(3):386–9. https://doi.org/10.1007/BF02981967. Available in: http://link.springer.com/10.1007/BF02981967.
92. Strauss PZ, Hamlin SK, Dang J. Tumor lysis syndrome: a unique solute disturbance. Nurs Clin N Am. 2017; https://doi.org/10.1016/j.cnur.2017.01.008.
93. Middeke JM, et al. Use of rasburicase in a pregnant woman with acute lymphoblastic leukaemia and imminent tumour lysis syndrome. Ann Hematol. 2014; https://doi.org/10.1007/s00277-013-1836-8.
94. Luzzatto L, Nannelli C, Notaro R. Glucose-6-phosphate dehydrogenase deficiency. Hematol Oncol Clin North Am. 2016; https://doi.org/10.1016/j.hoc.2015.11.006.
95. Shaikh SA, et al. Rational use of rasburicase for the treatment and management of tumor lysis syndrome. J Oncol Pharm Pract. 2018;24(3):176–84. https://doi.org/10.1177/107815521668 7152. Available in: http://journals.sagepub.com/doi/10.1177/1078155216687152.
96. Becker MA, et al. Febuxostat compared with allopurinol in patients with hyperuricemia and gout. N Engl J Med. 2005; https://doi.org/10.1056/NEJMoa050373.
97. Robinson PC, Dalbeth N. Febuxostat for the treatment of hyperuricaemia in gout. Expert Opin Pharmacother. 2018; https://doi.org/10.1080/14656566.2018.1498842.
98. Grewal HK, Martinez JR, Espinoza LR. Febuxostat: drug review and update. Expert Opin Drug Metab Toxicol. 2014;10(5):747–58. https://doi.org/10.1517/17425255.2014.904285. Available in: http://www.tandfonline.com/doi/full/10.1517/17425255.2014.904285.
99. Hussar DA, Bilbow C. New drugs: febuxostat, lacosamide, and rufinamide. J Am Pharm Assoc. 2009;49(3):460–3. https://doi.org/10.1331/JAPhA.2009.09516. Available in: https://linkinghub.elsevier.com/retrieve/pii/S1544319115310074.
100. Bellinghieri G, Santoro D, Savica V. Emerging drugs for hyperphosphatemia. Expert Opin Emerg Drugs. 2007; https://doi.org/10.1517/14728214.12.3.355.

101. Bellés M, et al. Effects of oral aluminum on essential trace elements metabolism during pregnancy. Biol Trace Elem Res. 2001; https://doi.org/10.1385/BTER:79:1:67.
102. Mahadevan U. Gastrointestinal medications in pregnancy. Best Pract Res Clin Gastroenterol. 2007; https://doi.org/10.1016/j.bpg.2007.06.002.
103. Rossignol P, et al. Emergency management of severe hyperkalemia: guideline for best practice and opportunities for the future. Pharmacol Res. 2016;113:585–91. https://doi.org/10.1016/j.phrs.2016.09.039. Available in: https://linkinghub.elsevier.com/retrieve/pii/S104366181630723X.
104. Hagan AE, et al. Sodium polystyrene sulfonate for the treatment of acute hyperkalemia: a retrospective study. Clin Nephrol. 2016; https://doi.org/10.5414/CN108628.
105. Tosi P, et al. Consensus conference on the management of tumor lysis syndrome. Haematologica. 2008;93(12):1877–85. https://doi.org/10.3324/haematol.13290.
106. Vázquez-Rodríguez JG. Hemodialysis and pregnancy: technical aspects. Cir Cir. 2010;78(1):99–102. Available in: http://www.ncbi.nlm.nih.gov/pubmed/20226136.
107. Koenig C, et al. Association of time to antibiotics and clinical outcomes in patients with fever and neutropenia during chemotherapy for cancer: a systematic review. Support Care Cancer. 2020;28:1369–83. https://doi.org/10.1007/s00520-019-04961-4.
108. Randhawa JK, Ferrajoli A. A review of supportive care and recommended preventive approaches for patients with chronic lymphocytic leukemia. Expert Rev Hematol. 2015; https://doi.org/10.1586/17474086.2016.1129893.
109. Hilal T, et al. Chronic lymphocytic leukemia and infection risk in the era of targeted therapies: linking mechanisms with infections. Blood Rev. 2018;32:387–99. https://doi.org/10.1016/j.blre.2018.03.004.
110. Cohen JB, Blum KA. Evaluation and management of lymphoma and leukemia in pregnancy. Clin Obstet Gynecol. 2011;54(4):556–66.
111. Azim HA Jr, et al. Treatment of the pregnant mother with cancer: a systematic review on the use of cytotoxic, endocrine, targeted agents and immunotherapy during pregnancy. Part II: Hematological tumors. Cancer Treat Rev. 2010;36:110–21. https://doi.org/10.1016/j.ctrv.2009.11.004.
112. Cottreau JM, Barr VO. A review of antiviral and antifungal use and safety during pregnancy. Pharmacotherapy. 2016;36(6):668–78. https://doi.org/10.1002/phar.1764.
113. Abadi U, et al. Leukemia and lymphoma in pregnancy. Hematol Oncol Clin N Am. 2011;25:277–91. https://doi.org/10.1016/j.hoc.2011.01.001.
114. National Comprehensive Cancer Network. Prevention and treatment of cancer related infections. (Version 1.2020). https://www.nccn.org/professionals/physician_gls/pdf/infections.pdf. Accessed 10 Mar 2020.
115. Pilmis B, et al. Antifungal drugs during pregnancy: an updated review. J Antimicrob Chemother. 2015;70:14–22. https://doi.org/10.1093/jac/dku355.
116. Vlachadis N, et al. Oral fluconazole during pregnancy and risk of birth defects. N Engl J Med. 2013;369:2061.
117. Chang CC, et al. New developments and directions in the clinical application of the Echinocandins. Arch Toxicol. 2017;91:1613–21. https://doi.org/10.1007/s00204-016-1916-3.
118. Mueller M, et al. A comparison of liposomal amphotericin B with sodium stibogluconate for the treatment of visceral leishmaniasis in pregnancy in Sudan. J Antimicrob Chemother. 2006;58(4):811–5.
119. Bitterman R, et al. Influenza vaccines in immunosuppressed adults with cancer (Review). Cochrane Database Syst Rev. 2018;(2):CD008983. https://doi.org/10.1002/14651858. CD008983.pub3.
120. Rogan SC, Beigi RH. Treatment of viral infections during pregnancy. Clin Perinatol. 2019;46:235–56. https://doi.org/10.1016/j.clp.2019.02.009.
121. Brzezińska-Wcislo L, et al. Pregnancy: a therapeutic dilemma. Adv Dermatol Allergol. 2017;34(5):433–8. https://doi.org/10.5114/ada.2017.71108.

122. Chen CY, et al. High risk of hepatitis B reactivation among patients with acute myeloid leukemia. PLoS One. 2015;10(5):e0126037. https://doi.org/10.1371/journal.pone.0126037.
123. Wu T, et al. Role of hepatitis B antibody in predicting reactivation of resolved hepatitis B virus infection in leukemia patients. Antivir Res. 2020;177:104765. https://doi.org/10.1016/j.antiviral.2020.104765.
124. Pan CQ, Lee HM. Antiviral therapy for chronic hepatitis B in pregnancy. Semin Liver Dis. 2013;33(2):138–46. https://doi.org/10.1055/s-0033-1345718.
125. Gu JX, et al. The detection of bacterial infections in leukemia patients using procalcitonin levels. Leuk Lymphoma. 2019; https://doi.org/10.1080/10428194.2019.1646906.
126. Gurman G. Pregnancy and successful labor in the course of chronic lymphocytic leukemia. Am J Hematol. 2002;71:208–10. https://doi.org/10.1002/ajh.10216.
127. Pejovic T, Schwartz PE. Leukemias. Clin Obstet Gynecol. 2002;45(3):866–78. https://doi.org/10.1097/01.grf.0000022391.03824.2d.
128. Muanda FT, et al. Use of antibiotics during pregnancy and risk of spontaneous abortion. CMAJ. 2017;17(189):E625–33. https://doi.org/10.1503/cmaj.161020.
129. Lamont HF, et al. Safety of antimicrobial treatment during pregnancy: a current review of resistance, immunomodulation and teratogenicity. Expert Opin Drug Saf. 2014; https://doi.org/10.1517/14740338.2014.939580.
130. Doi Y, Chambers HF. Penicillins and β-lactamase inhibitors. In: Mendell, Douglas and Bennetes's: basic principles in the diagnosis and management of infectious diseases. 8th ed., Cap. 20. Philadelphia: Elsevier/Saunders; 2015. p. 262–77.
131. Matuszkiewicz-Rowińsk J, et al. Urinary tract infections in pregnancy: old and new unresolved diagnostic and therapeutic problems. Arch Med Sci. 2015;11(1):67–77. https://doi.org/10.5114/aoms.2013.39202.
132. Forge A, Schacht J. Aminoglycoside antibiotics. Audiol Neurootol. 2000;5:3–22.
133. Aldred KJ, et al. Mechanism of quinolone action and resistance. Biochemistry. 2014;53:1565–74. https://doi.org/10.1021/bi5000564.
134. Bookstaver PB, et al. A review of antibiotic use in pregnancy. Pharmacotherapy. 2015;35(11):1052–62.
135. Mylonas I. Antibiotic chemotherapy during pregnancy and lactation period: aspects for consideration. Arch Gynecol Obstet. 2011;283:7–18. https://doi.org/10.1007/s00404-010-1646-3.
136. Lee JJ, Swain SM. Peripheral neuropathy induced by microtubule-stabilizing agents. J Clin Oncol. 2006;24(10):1633–42. https://doi.org/10.1200/JCO.2005.04.0543.
137. Mabie WC. Peripheral neuropathies during pregnancy. Clin Obstet Gynecol. 2005;48(1):57–66.
138. Addington J, Freimer M. Chemotherapy-induced peripheral neuropathy: an update on the current understanding. F1000Res. 2016;5:F1000. https://doi.org/10.12688/f1000research.8053.1.
139. Gustavson K, et al. Maternal fever during pregnancy and offspring attention deficit hyperactivity disorder. Sci Rep. 2019;9:9519. https://doi.org/10.1038/s41598-019-45920-7.
140. Rozovski U, et al. Targeting inflammatory pathways in chronic lymphocytic leukemia. Crit Rev Oncol Hematol. 2013; https://doi.org/10.1016/j.critrevonc.2013.07.011.
141. Nadeau-Vallée M, et al. Sterile inflammation and pregnancy complications: a review. Reproduction. 2016;152:277–92. https://doi.org/10.1530/REP-16-0453.
142. Shaulov A, et al. Pain in patients with newly diagnosed or relapsed acute leukemia. Support Care Cancer. 2019;27:2789–97. https://doi.org/10.1007/s00520-018-4583-5.
143. Ostensen ME, Skomsvoll JF. Anti-inflammatory pharmacotherapy during pregnancy. Expert Opin Pharmacother. 2004;5(3):571–80.
144. Li DK, et al. Exposure to non-steroidal anti-inflammatory drugs during pregnancy and risk of miscarriage: population based cohort study. BMJ. 2003;327(7411):368. https://doi.org/10.1136/bmj.327.7411.368.
145. Babb M, et al. Treating pain during pregnancy. Can Fam Physician. 2010;56(1):25, 27.

146. Dhanjal MK, Mitrou S. The obstetric care of the pregnant woman with cancer. In: Surbone A, et al., editors. Cancer and pregnancy. Cap. 17. Berlin, Heidelberg: Springer; 2008. p. 197–201.
147. Bloor M, et al. Nonsteroidal anti-inflammatory drugs during pregnancy and the initiation of lactation. Anesth Analg. 2013;116(5):1063–75. https://doi.org/10.1213/ANE.0b013e31828a4b54.
148. Padberg S. Safety of diclofenac use during early pregnancy: a prospectiveobservational cohort study. Reprod Toxicol. 2018;17:122–9. https://doi.org/10.1016/j.reprotox.2018.02.007.
149. Díaz RR, Rivera AL. Management of non-obstetric pain during pregnancy. Review article. Colomb J Anesthesiol. 2012;40(3):213–23.
150. Bandoli G, et al. A review of systemic corticosteroid use in pregnancy and the risk of select pregnancy and birth outcomes. Rheum Dis Clin N Am. 2017;43:489–502. https://doi.org/10.1016/j.rdc.2017.04.013.
151. Broussard CS, et al. Maternal treatment with opioid analgesics and risk for birth defects. Am J Obstet Gynecol. 2011;204(4):314.e1–11. https://doi.org/10.1016/j.ajog.2010.12.039. Epub 2011 Feb 23.
152. Kallen B, Reis M. Ongoing pharmacological management of chronic pain in pregnancy. Drugs. 2016;76(9):915–24. https://doi.org/10.1007/s40265-016-0582-3.
153. Yazdy MM, et al. Prescription opioids in pregnancy and birth outcomes: a review of the literature. J Pediatr Genet. 2015;4(2):58–70. https://doi.org/10.1055/s-0035-1556740.
154. Leppert W, Buss T. The role of corticosteroids in the treatment of pain in cancer patients. Curr Pain Headache Rep. 2012;16:307–13. https://doi.org/10.1007/s11916-012-0273-z.
155. Kemp MW, et al. The clinical use of corticosteroids in pregnancy. Hum Reprod Update. 2016;22(2):240–59. https://doi.org/10.1093/humupd/dmv047.
156. Zaghw A, et al. Pain management for pregnant women in the opioid crisis era. In: Shalik NA, editor. Pain management in special circumstances. London: IntechOpen; 2018. https://doi.org/10.5772/intechopen.79333.
157. Wang XS, et al. Clinical factors associated with cancer-related fatigue in patients being treated for leukemia and non-Hodgkin's lymphoma. J Clin Oncol. 2002;20(5):1319–28. https://doi.org/10.1200/JCO.2002.20.5.1319.
158. Chien LY, Ko YL. Fatigue during pregnancy predicts caesarean deliveries. J Adv Nurs. 2004;45(5):487–94. https://doi.org/10.1046/j.1365-2648.2003.02931.x.
159. Miller AH, et al. Acute leukemia masquerading as fatigue and anemia of pregnancy: a case report. Ann Clin Case Rep. 2016;1:1105.
160. Bialobok KM, Monga M. Fatigue and work in pregnancy. Curr Opin Obstet Gynecol. 2000;12(6):497–500. https://doi.org/10.1097/00001703-200012000-00007.
161. National Comprehensive Cancer Network. Cancer-related fatigue. (Version 1.2020). https://www.nccn.org/store/login/login.aspx?ReturnURL=https://www.nccn.org/professionals/physician_gls/pdf/fatigue.pdf. Accessed 21 Feb 2020.
162. Borodulin K, et al. Physical activity patterns during pregnancy. Med Sci Sports Exerc. 2008;40(11):1901–8. https://doi.org/10.1249/MSS.0b013e31817f1957.
163. Dimeo F, et al. Effects of endurance training on the physical performance of patients with hematological malignancies during chemotherapy. Support Care Cancer. 2003;11:623–8. https://doi.org/10.1007/s00520-003-0512-2.
164. Pottegard A, et al. First-trimester exposure to methylphenidate: a population-based cohort study. J Clin Psychiatry. 2014;75(1):88–93. https://doi.org/10.4088/JCP.13m08708.
165. Hoque R, Chesson AL Jr. Conception, pregnancy, delivery, and breastfeeding in a narcoleptic patient with cataplexy. J Clin Sleep Med. 2008;4(6):601–3.
166. World Health Organization. Anaemia. https://www.who.int/health-topics/anaemia#tab=tab_1. Access in 04/2020.
167. Annamraju H, Pavord S. Anaemia in pregnancy. Br J Hosp Med. 2016;77(10):584–8.
168. Jimenez K, Kulnigg-Dabsch S, Gasche C. Management of iron deficiency anemia. Gastroenterol Hepatol. 2015;11(4):241–50.

169. Waller D, Sampson T. Anaemia and haematopoietic colony stimulating factors, Chapter 47. In: Medical pharmacology and therapeutics. 5th ed. Edinburgh: Elsevier; 2018. p. 537–45.
170. Royal College of Obstetricians and Gynaecologists. Blood transfusion in obstetrics green-top guideline no. 47, May 2015.
171. American Pregnancy Association. Blood transfusions during pregnancy. https://americanpregnancy.org/pregnancy-concerns/blood-transfusions-during-pregnancy/. Access in 04/2020.
172. Diamantidis MD, et al. Iron chelation therapy of transfusion-dependent β-thalassemia during pregnancy in the era of novel drugs: is deferasirox toxic? Int J Hematol. 2016;103(5):537–44.
173. Piccioni MG, et al. Use of deferoxamine (DFO) in transfusion-dependent b-thalassemia during pregnancy: a retrospective study. Taiwanese J Obstet Gynecol. 2020;59:120–2.
174. Beeley L. Adverse effects of drugs in the first trimester of pregnancy. Clin Obstet Gynaecol. 1986;13:177–95.
175. Sifakis S, et al. Erythropoietin in the treatment of iron deficiency anemia during pregnancy. Gynecol Obstet Invest. 2001;51:150–6.
176. Breymann C, Visca E, Huch R, Huch A. Efficacy and safety of intravenously administered iron sucrose with and without adjuvant recombinant human erythropoietin for the treatment of resistant iron-deficiency anemia during pregnancy. Am J Obstet Gynecol. 2001;184(4):662–7.
177. Ifeanyi OE, Uzoma OG. A review on erythropietin in pregnancy. J Gynecol Women's Health. 2018;8(3):555740.
178. Body C, Christie JA. Gastrointestinal diseases in pregnancy. Gastroenterol Clin North Am. 2016;45:267–83.
179. Giorgi F, et al. Pathophysiology of gastro-oesophageal reflux disease. ACTA Otorhinolaryngol Ital. 2006;26:241–6.
180. Ali RAR, Egan LJ. Gastroesophageal reflux disease in pregnancy. Best Pract Res Clin Gastroenterol. 2007;21(5):793–806.
181. Gomes CF, et al. Gastrointestinal diseases during pregnancy: what does the gastroenterologist need to know? Ann Gastroenterol. 2018;31:385–94.
182. Ching C, Lam S. Antacids: indications and limitations. Drugs. 1994;47:305–17.
183. Richter JE. Heartburn, nausea, and vomiting during pregnancy. In: Pregnancy in gastrointestinal disorders. Bethesda: ACG Monograph American College of Physicians; 2007. p. 18–25.
184. Briggs GG, Freeman RY, Yaffe SJ. Drugs in pregnancy and lactation: a reference guide to foetal and neonatal risk. Baltimore: William and Wilkins; 2002.

Chapter 10
Breastfeeding During Chemotherapy Treatment for Leukemia

Carolina Witchmichen Penteado Schmidt

As a general rule, breastfeeding is not recommended during chemotherapy treatment. The patient is generally advised to interrupt breastfeeding during systemic chemotherapy treatment for fear of serious adverse effects on the neonate. However, there is a lack of information published on this issue, and few studies have evaluated the safety of breastfeeding during or after chemotherapy; the excretion of a drug in human milk guides this decision [1–3].

Women who receive chemotherapy during pregnancy are more likely to have difficulties breastfeeding, presenting a decreased breast milk supply and needing to provide supplemental feeding to their neonates or infants. A study showed no significant difference in maternal age, cancer type, or stage regarding breastfeeding difficulties among women who received chemotherapy. However, gestational age at the first cycle and the number of cycles were significant factors. Antepartum and postpartum depression was not associated with decreased breast milk production [1, 2].

There is an increased rate of women diagnosed with cancer during pregnancy and lactation. Probably, that occurs due to the rising incidence of pregnancy in older age. It is well known that breastfeeding is essential to improve neonates and infants' health, including their cognitive development. Breastfeeding is an essential physiologic process not only to provide nutrition but also to protect the child against infection and immunologic disorders. Bioactive agents that are present in human milk promote the development of a newborn's host defense system and the maturation of the gastrointestinal tract. A large meta-analysis showed a reduced risk of testicular, gastric, and pre-menopausal breast cancer in adults who had been breastfed. Studies showed that breastfeeding mothers, principally those younger than 30 years, have a lower risk of developing breast cancer. The reduced risk of ovarian cancer development was also related to breastfeeding women [1, 2].

C. W. P. Schmidt (✉)
Pediatric Oncology Pharmacist & Scientific Writer, Curitiba, Paraná, Brazil

© Springer Nature Switzerland AG 2021
C. W. P. Schmidt, K. M. Otoni (eds.), *Chemotherapy and Pharmacology for Leukemia in Pregnancy*, https://doi.org/10.1007/978-3-030-54058-6_10

181

10.1   Excretion of Drugs into Human Milk

We should remember that patients who undergo chemotherapy for leukemia also receive many other supportive drugs, as well as drugs to treat infections and other transitory conditions. The excretion of drugs into milk depends upon several characteristics of the drug, such as lipid solubility, molecular size, ionization, concentration and half-life in maternal plasma, and protein binding. The breastfeeding phase also matters. Plasma to milk transfer is highest during the first week of breastfeeding because of the presence of larger gaps between the alveolar breast cells. The same might be true during the last period of breastfeeding, when glandular involution occurs and the amount of milk decreases. Large molecules, which are usually segregated into mother's plasma, may be found in milk during these phases [2].

The maternal plasma level of each specific drug is the most crucial factor in determining the concentration of drug transferred into breast milk. However, high lipid solubility and low molecular weight of a drug may favor its passage through breast milk by simple diffusion, and it is not concentration-dependent. Large molecules with high molecular weight (P600 Daltons), such as monoclonal antibodies and heparin, can hardly penetrate human milk. Drugs with high albumin-bound fractions can be present in lesser quantities in human milk than drugs with a high free plasma fraction. The relatively low pH of human milk (7.0–7.2) favors the accumulation of weakly basic drugs [2].

If a drug is present in milk, the risks of toxicity for the neonates and infants depend on the volume of milk received, oral bioavailability of the drug, and neonatal pharmacodynamics. Some drugs may have a local effect on the infant's gastrointestinal tract, and this should also be considered [2].

10.2   Lactogenesis

Ductal development occurs during puberty; later, proliferative lobular development occurs during the luteal phases of the menstrual cycle. In the period of early pregnancy, alveolar development starts with milk-secreting units. Then, lactogenesis occurs during mid-pregnancy stage; its first stage is the secretory differentiation, in which the mammary epithelial cells differentiate into lactocytes (secretory mammary epithelial cells) with the capacity to synthesize lactose, casein, a-lactalbumin, and fatty acids. That stage is mediated by progesterone, prolactin, and human placental lactogen. During mid-pregnancy, extensive lobular clusters are formed and the development continues until parturition. Studies showed that 75% of women who started treatment with chemotherapy at 17 weeks of gestation, just before or during lactogenesis stage I, presented decreased or no breast milk production. After that, lactogenesis II occurs, which is also called secretory activation. During this stage, milk secretion is activated and occurs at about the time of parturition, mediated by progesterone. Increased synthesis occurs by mammary lactocytes of milk components, such as lactose and citrate. Milk is produced in copious amounts during the lactogenesis II period and in the first 4 days postpartum. Patients perceive milk coming by 40 h postpartum or after. A delay in the onset of lactogenesis II affects subsequent lactation. Mothers of preterm infants are more likely to have problems at the stage of lactogenesis II as a result of stress, maternal illness, operative delivery, or antenatal pharmacologic therapies. Studies showed that mothers of preterm express significantly lower volumes of milk, which seems to be nonrelated to prolactin and occurs even at day 10 postpartum [1].

Histological evaluation showed lobular atrophy with associated lymphoplasmacytic infiltrates and fibrosis in patients who received neoadjuvant chemotherapy during pregnancy, suggesting that chemotherapy may damage the acinar cells of breast lobules. The lactation changes shown in pathology specimens support patients' reports that breast milk production is decreased after chemotherapy [1].

Maternal stress and fetal stress are associated with impaired lactogenesis. Acute physical and mental stress can impair milk ejection reflux due to a change in the release of oxytocin. If this occurs repeatedly, it could reduce milk production [1].

10.3   Guidelines on Breastfeeding During or After Chemotherapy Treatment for Leukemia

Patients who do not require chemotherapy after parturition may be able to breastfeed. The number of reports detailing the measurement of chemotherapeutic agents in breast milk is limited. Nevertheless, even if chemotherapy drugs are excreted into breast milk, the infant's toxicity, if any, depends on the absorbed volume of milk, the oral bioavailability of the drug itself, and the neonate's pharmacokinetics [1].

In all cases evaluated in a study, at least seven full half-lives after the last chemotherapy occurred before delivery and breastfeeding. Only 33.8% of women who attempted breastfeeding after receiving chemotherapy 3 weeks before delivery were able to breastfeed their newborn successfully, and 65% had minimal or no milk production. Earlier gestational age at the first treatment and the number of cycles received during pregnancy were significantly related to decreased milk production [1].

The golden standard is direct sampling and pharmacokinetic measurement of the drugs and their metabolites in the milk. Variations in individual metabolism may be particularly relevant in cancer patients when impairment in renal and hepatic functions is observed [1].

The type of cancer, stage, maternal age, depression, gestational age at the last chemotherapy, and the number of days between chemotherapy completion and delivery did not significantly affect breastfeeding success. Due to the well-known decreased breast milk production after chemotherapy, patients should be warned about the likelihood of decreased or no breast milk production [1].

10.4   Experiences of Patients

A telephone follow-up study to evaluate the capacity to breastfeed after chemotherapy was conducted with 74 women. These women received chemotherapy during the second or third trimester of pregnancy. Thirty-four percent of these women were able to breastfeed their infants exclusively. Sixty-four percent of women reported breastfeeding difficulties. Women who received cancer diagnosis during pregnancy but did not receive chemotherapy had 91% breastfeeding success rate (22 mothers). There were some statistically significant correlations; one of them was the number of cycles: in general, mothers with an average of 5.5 cycles of chemotherapy had breastfeeding difficulties, and mothers who had 3.8 cycles had no difficulties. Pregnancy time also made a difference: mothers who said they had breastfeeding difficulties received their first cycle of chemotherapy on an average of 3.4 weeks earlier in pregnancy [9].

10.5   Microbiota of the Milk After Chemotherapy

The neonatal gut is not mature and starts to develop its microbiota with human milk, which is an essential source of bacteria for the developing infant. It is estimated that a 1-year-old infant has a mature intestine, which enables them to consume foods like honey because spores of *Clostridium botulinum* can be present in the honey and cause infant botulism. A mature gut has bacteria that compete with the spores and do not let them develop into active bacteria.

Human milk is also an important source of nutrients, influencing not only bacterial composition but also the host directly. A study was carried out with milk collected every 2 weeks over 4 months from a woman undergoing chemotherapy for Hodgkin's lymphoma, and it was compared with milk collected from a healthy woman. Microbial profiles were analyzed by 16S sequencing and the metabolome by mass spectrometry. Chemotherapy caused a significant deviation from a healthy microbial and metabolomic profile, presenting depletion of *Bifidobacterium*, *Eubacterium*, *Staphylococcus,* and *Cloacibacterium* in favor of *Acinetobacter*, Xanthomonadaceae, and *Stenotrophomonas*. The metabolites docosahexaenoic acid and inositol, which are known for their beneficial effects, were decreased. Since human milk is important to develop immunity and colonization of the neonatal gut, it is important to evaluate not only the presence of chemotherapeutic agents in milk but also its quality regarding bacteria. The bacteria acquired during infancy also have an influence later in life on disease risk and play a major role in determining the composition of the adult gut microbiome. In addition to the gut microbiota, human milk also plays a role in the synthesis of metabolites, such as fatty acids, carbohydrates, proteins, and vitamins, which are important not only for infant development but also long-term health [10].

10.6 Chemotherapeutic Agents in Milk

Pharmaceutical agents are prescribed for many women for various reasons after delivery. While many drugs, including most of the antibiotics, are not contraindicated during breastfeeding, when it comes to chemotherapeutics, the recommendation is that breastfeeding should be avoided until the drug has been cleared from the milk. That is the most sensate decision, since there are few available data on the passage of chemotherapeutic agents into human milk, and they do not affirm the same. There is a suggestion that antimetabolites—except for high-dose methotrexate—appear to be relatively safe. Anthracyclines and alkylating agents, including platinum compounds, should be avoided [2, 10]. However, there are lots of controversies between the information available. Some studies suggest some drugs are compatible with breastfeeding, while others suggest the same drugs are not.

10.6.1 Cytarabine

It is not known whether cytarabine is excreted in milk.

10.6.2 Daunorubicin

Although there are few studies about treatments with daunorubicin during pregnancy, there are some reports of its use during pregnancy. It is recommended not to breastfeed during or immediately after the treatment with daunorubicin since it is unknown if it is excreted into milk. Moreover, there is no sufficient amount of reliable data about breastfeeding and daunorubicin dosage in milk. Breastfeeding is also contraindicated for mothers who receive liposomal daunorubicin, which is a pregnancy risk-factor D. It is unknown if liposomal daunorubicin is excreted into the milk similar to the conventional daunorubicin [8].

10.6.3 Doxorubicin

As described in Chap. 2, doxorubicin can be used as an alternative treatment in patients who refuse to receive a medical termination of pregnancy, such as in the 7 + 3 AML protocol. Breastfeeding should not be performed by patients receiving doxorubicin. This drug can be detected in human milk at high levels, including its active metabolite doxorubicinol, for at least 72 h after exposure. Twenty-four hours after treatment with 70 mg/m^2 of doxorubicin IV—in association with cisplatin to treat ovarian cancer—it was found in significant levels in the form of doxorubicin and doxorubicinol in milk (128 and 111 μg/L, respectively). The maximum concentration of doxorubicin in milk was found to be 4.4 times higher than the concentration detected in concomitant plasma samples. The AUC (area under the curve) of doxorubicinol was ten times higher in milk than in plasma. If a neonate or an infant receives their mother's milk throughout the 72 h after doxorubicin administration, the baby would have received an estimated 2% of maternal weight-adjusted dosage [2].

10.6.4 Cyclophosphamide

Cases of serious adverse reactions in children fed by mothers receiving cyclophosphamide were reported. In one reported case, the mother received six cycles of weekly administrations of 800 mg IV cyclophosphamide and 2 mg vincristine, as well as daily oral prednisolone at a dosage of 30 mg/m^2. Her four-month-old child presented neutropenia 9 days after her mother's last dose of chemotherapy. The contribution of vincristine cannot be excluded; however, the neutropenia was reported as caused by cyclophosphamide. In another reported case, a breastfeeding woman received 6 mg/kg/day IV cyclophosphamide. Her 23-day-old child presented neutropenia, thrombocytopenia, and low hemoglobin level after 3 days. There is no data about the estimated quantity of cyclophosphamide in milk reported in those two cases.

10.6.5 Cytarabine

It is not known if cytarabine is excreted in milk [8].

10.6.6 Etoposide

A patient who received five daily doses of IV etoposide 80 mg/m^2 , as well as mitoxantrone and cytarabine for promyelocytic leukemia had her milk evaluated. Etoposide milk levels reached peaks of about 600, 580, and 800 μg/L immediately after the last three doses, respectively. Etoposide was undetectable in her milk 24 h after each dose. Another mother received five daily doses of etoposide 80 mg/m^2 and cytarabine 170 mg/m^2 intravenously plus three daily doses of mitoxantrone 6 mg/m^2 intravenously. She breastfed her infant 3 weeks after the third dose of mitoxantrone, at a time when mitoxantrone was still detectable in milk, but the infant had no apparent abnormalities at 16 months of age. Reported data indicates that it is probably safe to breastfeed 72 h after the administration of etoposide. The concentration of etoposide in milk reached a peak after the third dose and then dramatically dropped until it was undetectable in milk after 24 h. Although they are single reports, it seems reasonable to wait at least 72 h after etoposide administration [9].

10.6.7 Imatinib and Sunitinib

Human milk was collected and evaluated in three pregnant patients with chronic myeloid leukemia who received treatment with imatinib 400 mg/day. A high concentration of imatinib and its active metabolite CGP74588 were detected in a single sample of human milk, which was collected 7 days postpartum and 15 h after a 400 mg oral dose of imatinib (596 ng/mL and 1513 ng/mL, respectively). Although an infant consuming 600–1000 mL of milk daily would ingest only 1.2–2.0 mg of both molecules, the authors of the study concluded that breastfeeding should be avoided by nursing patients being treated with imatinib because of concerns regarding abnormal growth of the peripheral microvasculature and nervous system of the baby due to the inhibition of platelet-derived growth factor receptor β (PDGFRβ). Similar results were obtained in breast milk samples collected over 2 months from another CML (chronic myeloid leukemia) patient who had been breastfeeding her son during her treatment with imatinib at 400 mg/day. Imatinib and CGP74588 showed relatively high concentrations in milk, and the milk-plasma ratios were found to be 0.5 and 0.9, respectively. Considering the maximum daily milk intake of 777 mL, the infant would have received no more than 3 mg/day of imatinib and its metabolite GCP74588, which is not near to the therapeutic ranges. Another study reported that imatinib was detected in several milk samples collected on different postpartum days [9].

Animal reproductive studies have shown that sunitinib and its metabolites were extensively excreted in milk at concentrations up to 12 times higher than those in plasma [9].

10.6.8 Methotrexate

Although there are many concerns about methotrexate and it is contraindicated during pregnancy, it has been studied in human milk. The concentration of methotrexate in milk was evaluated for 12 consecutive days in one breastfeeding woman with choriocarcinoma. She received oral doses of 22.5 mg/day. A peak milk level of 2.3 µg/L occurred 10 h after drug administration; then a drop in the concentration occurred with a milk/plasma ratio of 0.08. Another woman, who received an intramuscular dose of 65 mg of methotrexate for ectopic pregnancy had six samples collected over 24 h. Methotrexate was undetectable in all milk samples. Patients treated with low doses of methotrexate for arthritis (up to 65 mg) can be allowed to breastfeed, but not all professionals agree with that. Methotrexate is administered from very low doses to extremely high doses, and only the lowest doses can be undetected or almost undetected. When medium- or high-dose methotrexate is administered, the passage into milk is likely to occur, and potential adverse effects in the neonate or infant may not be excluded. This can be similar to the neonate or infant having an oral dose of methotrexate, since about 33% of the dose present in milk can be absorbed. Oral methotrexate may cause gut inflammation in the infant. Thus, it is probably safer to discard the milk for at least a week after methotrexate administration in breastfeeding women [2].

10.6.9 Mitoxantrone

Mitoxantrone enters the milk and also presents slow clearance. A woman received etoposide, cytarabine, and mitoxantrone for acute promyelocytic leukemia. The patient underwent chemotherapy with daily doses of IV mitoxantrone 6 mg/m^2 for 3 days, daily doses of IV etoposide 80 mg/m^2 for 5 days, and intravenous cytarabine 170 mg/m^2. Very slow clearance of mitoxantrone was demonstrated. Its level decreased gradually and reached a plateau value of 20 µg/L by 7 days. It remained at 18 µg/L at 28 days after the last dose. Although it is a single report, it seems reasonable not to breastfeed while on treatment with mitoxantrone [9].

10.6.10 Triple Intrathecal Chemotherapy

Triple intrathecal chemotherapy with methotrexate, cytarabine, and a corticosteroid drug (either dexamethasone or prednisolone) is used to treat meningeal leukemia. The triple intrathecal chemotherapy should be handled by an experienced oncology pharmacist only. Intrathecal methotrexate must not be used before 28 weeks of gestation. If the mother opts against strongly recommended pregnancy termination, intrathecal methotrexate can be replaced by intrathecal hydrocortisone and cytarabine, which are pregnancy risk-category D drugs, and the benefit justifies the risk to the fetus [11].

With intrathecal administration, levels of cytarabine in the cerebrospinal fluid declined with the first-order half-life of about 2 h, and little conversion to uracil arabinoside (ara-U) was observed since cerebrospinal fluid levels of deaminase are low. Cerebrospinal fluid levels of cytarabine are lower than plasma levels after intravenous injection. However, one patient in whom cerebrospinal fluid levels were examined after 2 h of constant intravenous infusion approached 40% of the steady-state plasma level. With intrathecal administration, levels of cytarabine in the cerebrospinal fluid declined with the first-order half-life of about 2 h. It is unknown whether cytarabine is excreted in milk either for intrathecal or intravenous administration. Intrathecal doses are much lower than intravenous doses; however, it is not known whether cytarabine and its metabolites can be present in the milk after an intrathecal administration [8, 12].

Both prednisolone and dexamethasone diffuse rapidly out of the central nervous system (CSF) [13].

10.7 Supportive Drugs

10.7.1 Granulocyte Colony-Stimulating Factor

The granulocyte colony-stimulating factor (G-CSF) filgrastim was measured in the milk of a nursing woman who received 300–600 µg of the drug for peripheral blood hematopoietic stem cell harvesting. Filgrastim was detected in the milk at a dosage of 188 ng/L 22 h after the first administration; the concentration slowly decreased and was undetectable at <10 ng/L 70 h after the last administration. Filgrastim is not orally absorbed, and any quantity excreted into milk is unlikely to adversely affect the child [2].

Human milk contains significant levels of G-CSF, and the concentration increases after intra-amniotic infection and during the first 2 postpartum days. A breastfeeding woman receiving the recombinant G-CSF lenograstim in doses of 300–600 µg to be a donor for a peripheral blood hematopoietic stem cell transplantation. Presented lenograstim milk levels increased during therapy up to 85.7 ng/L on day 6, which can be an infant dosage of about 0.013 µg/kg [2].

10.7.2 Antiemetics

10.7.2.1 Ondansetron

Serotonin (5-HT) receptor subtype-3 antagonists, such as ondansetron, antagonize the emetic effects of serotonin in the small bowel, vagus nerve, and chemoreceptor trigger zone (CTZ). They are effective for chemotherapy nausea, are safe from the pharmacological point of view, and have few side effects—the most common adverse effects are headache and gastrointestinal symptoms, including diarrhea. There is not a sufficient amount of data published on ondansetron related to breastfeeding. However, a randomized, double-blind study compared placebo to ondansetron (4 mg given IV after cesarean), and there was no difference in the time of the first breastfeeding between the two groups. The conclusion was that this drug appears not to affect the onset of breastfeeding. No adverse effects have been reported in neonates and infants being breastfed by mothers receiving ondansetron. Ondansetron has been used in infants, and it is challenging to substitute ondansetron since it is the most used drug for nausea in oncology and hematology [4, 5].

10.7.2.2 Metoclopramide

Metoclopramide is not the first choice for nausea due to chemotherapy, in part because of its contraindications, such as those for people susceptible to extrapyramidal effects, and mothers with a history of major depression—since there are indications that metoclopramide should probably be avoided in these women and not used for prolonged periods in any mothers during this time of high susceptibility. Metoclopramide is still largely used for delayed nausea and vomiting. Metoclopramide is excreted in breastmilk. The dose received by neonates or infants may vary; some receive less than 10% of the maternal weight-adjusted dosage, while others receive doses that achieve pharmacologically active serum levels, as well as elevated serum prolactin. There could be a possible gastrointestinal side effect in neonates or infants receiving milk with metoclopramide. Most studies have not found adverse effects in breastfed neonates and infants during maternal metoclopramide use, but there is a claim that many of them did not adequately observe the side effects [6, 7].

It is contraindicated to prescribe metoclopramide for children younger than 1 year. And it should only be used as a second-line option for the prevention of delayed chemotherapy-induced nausea and vomiting, as well as for treatment of established postoperative nausea and vomiting. Since ondansetron is used in infants and no adverse effects have been reported in neonates and infants being breastfed by mothers receiving ondansetron, it is a better choice than metoclopramide [4–7].
Metoclopramide increases serum prolactin and has been studied and used to increase milk supply. A meta-analysis of five studies with metoclopramide versus placebo concluded 3 weeks of metoclopramide administration could increase prolactin and that only 2 weeks cannot. There is no consensus about the efficacy of metoclopramide in increasing milk supply, and its use to increase the milk is questionable. Prophylactic use of metoclopramide to increase the milk of mothers of preterm neonates has shown little or no benefit [6, 7].

10.7.3   Pain Management

Morphine, codeine, and acetaminophen are considered compatible with breastfeeding [15].

Morphine is often used for pain management during cancer treatments because of its efficacy and the possibility of using it without too many concerns regarding drug interactions. Although reproductive studies describing the use of narcotic analgesics in human pregnancies are limited, these drugs have been used in therapeutic doses by pregnant patients for many years and have not been linked to the elevated risk of malformations. Morphine is excreted in breast milk in low concentrations. In a study with pregnant patients who received morphine either via epidural, intravenous, or intramuscular routes, the highest level was found in the milk half an hour after giving the drug. The highest level was 0.082 mg per liter of milk when administered by the epidural route and 0.5 mg per liter of milk when given intravenously or intramuscularly. The mean M/P ratio was 2.45. If morphine is given orally, it presents a low bioavailability and tends not to be present in high amounts in the milk, being compatible with breastfeeding. Even though the neonate or infant receives a small amount of the drug, morphine has been used for managing pain in neonates and infants for years [15–18].

Only 0.04–0.23% of the maternal dose of acetaminophen is excreted in breast milk. The peak level of acetaminophen is observed 1–2 h after ingestion, and its half-life in milk is less comparable to that in plasma, which is 1.35–3.5 h (mean 2.7 h) [15].

10.7.4 Nonsteroidal Anti-inflammatories

The amount of nonsteroidal anti-inflammatories (NSAIDs) in the milk tends to be minimum. Ibuprofen and diclofenac were below the level of detection [15]. However, naproxen does not seem to be safe. It appears minimally in breast milk with an M/P ratio of 0.01, but it presents a long half-life. One 7-day-old infant developed hematuria, prolonged gastrointestinal bleeding, and acute anemia while his mother was treated with naproxen [15].

10.7.5 Antibiotics, Antifungals, Antimalarials, and Anthelmintics

Although there is little information about the presence of chemotherapeutic agents in milk, the presence of antibiotics in milk is a subject that has been studied extensively. There are three mechanisms of antibiotic passage to the milk: passive diffusion across a concentration gradient, active transport against a concentration gradient, and transcellular diffusion [19].

It has to be considered when the mother is on short- or long-term antibiotic therapy. Based on pharmacokinetics and case reports published, it is now possible to determine the effects of several maternal antibiotics on neonates and infants. It may be possible to minimize babies' exposure to untoward effects of antibiotics through awareness, prescription, and modifications in the antibiotic schedule. These issues need consideration in order to enable physicians and mothers to make the best possible decision for the baby [19].

Antibiotics and the risks for the baby during breastfeeding:

- The antibiotics that are safe for administration during breastfeeding are aminoglycosides, amoxycillin, amoxycillin/clavulanate, antitubercular drugs, cephalosporins, macrolides, and trimethoprim/sulphamethoxazole.
- The antibiotics with unknown effects during breastfeeding and/or should be used with caution are chloramphenicol, clindamycin, dapsone, mandelic acid, low-dose metronidazole, nalidixic acid, nitrofurantoin, penicillins, and tetracyclines.
- The antibiotics that are not compatible with breastfeeding are metronidazole (single high dose) and quinolones [19].

Antifungals and the risks for the baby during breastfeeding:

- The antifungal that is safe for administration during breastfeeding is ketoconazole.
- The antifungals with unknown effects during breastfeeding are amphotericin, fluconazole, flucytosine, and itraconazole.

Antimalarials and the risks for the baby during breastfeeding:

- The antimalarials safe for administration during breastfeeding are chloroquine, hydroxychloroquine, and quinine.
- The antimalarials with unknown effects during breastfeeding are mefloquine, pentamidine, proguanil, primaquine, and pyrimethamine.

Anthelminthic drugs and the risks for the baby during breastfeeding:
The effects of anthelminthic drugs on the baby after being breastfed by a mother being treated are not known, including mebendazole, pyrantel pamoate, praziquantel, quinacrine antihelminth, thiabendazole, and piperazine [19].

10.8 Big Picture of Chemotherapy and Breastfeeding

There are few studies about the presence of chemotherapeutic agents in milk and even less about their effect in neonates and nursery infants. There is a high variation between drugs in the concentration of chemotherapeutic agents and their active metabolites in human milk, as well as the dose-independent effects of these drugs. The effects of chemotherapy in the milk are not well described yet. Although it is not clear how much toxicity can be attributed to these drugs with regard to the baby during lactation, most researchers recommend avoiding breastfeeding until at least 2 weeks following the completion of chemotherapy. Sociocultural aspects may also be considered before making the decision [14, 19].

References

1. Stopenski S, Aslam A, Zhang X, Cardonick E. After chemotherapy treatment for maternal cancer during pregnancy, is breastfeeding possible? Breastfeed Med. 2017. https://link.springer.com/article/10.1007/s00404-008-0861-7.
2. Pistilli B, Bellettini G, Giovannetti E, et al. Chemotherapy, targeted agents, antiemetics and growth-factors in human milk: how should we counsel cancer patients about breastfeeding? Cancer Treat Rev. 2013;39:207–11.
3. Stopenski S, Aslam A, Zhang X, Cardonick E. After chemotherapy treatment for maternal cancer during pregnancy, is breastfeeding possible? Breastfeed Med. 2017;12(2):91–7. http://www.cancerandpregnancy.com/wp-content/uploads/2019/08/Breastfeeding-after-Chemotherapy-treatment-1.pdf.

4. Griffiths JD, Gyte GM, Paranjothy S, Brown HC, Broughton HK, Thomas J. Interventions for preventing nausea and vomiting in women undergoing regional anaesthesia for caesarean section. Cochrane Database Syst Rev. 2012;9(9):CD007579.
5. Ondansetron. LactMed: drugs and lactation database. Bethesda: National Library of Medicine (US). [Updated 2019 Feb 7]. https://www.ncbi.nlm.nih.gov/books/NBK500798/.
6. Metoclopramide. LactMed:drugs and lactation database. Bethesda: National Library of Medicine (US). [Updated 2018 Oct 31]. https://www.ncbi.nlm.nih.gov/books/NBK501352/.
7. European Medicines Agency. European Medicines Agency recommends changes to the use of metoclopramide. 2013. https://www.ema.europa.eu/en/documents/press-release/european-medicines-agency-recommends-changes-use-metoclopramide_en.pdf.
8. Bragalode DL. Drug information handbook for oncology. 13th ed. Hudson: Lexicomp; 2015.
9. Etoposide. LactMed: drugs and lactation database. Bethesda: National Library of Medicine. https://www.ncbi.nlm.nih.gov/books/NBK500643/.
10. Urbaniak C, McMillan A, Angelini M, et al. Effect of chemotherapy on the microbiota and metabolome of human milk, a case report. Micobiome. 2014;2:24. https://microbiomejournal.biomedcentral.com/articles/10.1186/2049-2618-2-24.
11. Zaidi A, Johnson LM, Church CL. Management of current pregnancy and acute lymphoblastic malignancy in teenaged patients: two illustrative cases and review of the literature. J Adolesc Young Adult Oncol. 2014;3(4):160–75.
12. Pfizer: Cytarabine. Label. http://labeling.pfizer.com/ShowLabeling.aspx?id=4398.
13. Balis FM, Lester CM, Chrousos GP, Heideman RL, Poplack DG. Differences in cerebrospinal fluid penetration of corticosteroids: possible relation to the prevention of meningeal leukemia. J Clin Oncol. 1987;5(2):202–7.
14. Shapira T, Pereg D, Lishner M. How I treat acute and chronic leukemia in pregnancy. Blood Rev. 2008;22:247–59.
15. Bar-Oz B, Bulkowstein M, Benyamini L, et al. Use of antibiotic and analgesic drugs during lactation. Drug-Safety. 2003;26:925–35.
16. Schmidt CWP. Chemotherapy in neonates and infants: pharmacological oncology for children under 1 year old. Cham: Springer; 2018.
17. Babb M, Koren G, Einarson A. Treating pain during pregnancy. Can Fam Physician. 2010;56(1):25, 27.
18. Kart T, Christrup LL, Rasmussen M. Recommended use of morphine in neonates, infants and children based on a literature review: part 2–clinical use. Paediatr Anaesth. 2008;7(2):93–101.
19. Mathew JL. Effect of maternal antibiotics on breast feeding infants. Postgrad Med J. 2004;80:196–200.

Chapter 11
Palliative Care for Patients with Leukemia During Pregnancy

Andrea Maria Novaes Machado and Polianna Mara Rodrigues de Souza

Cancer is a relevant public health problem, a disease of high incidence and prevalence, affecting individuals of all age groups. The World Health Organization (WHO) estimates that around 14 million new cases and approximately 8 million cancer deaths occur annually worldwide [1].

Although not a common occurrence, cancer can be diagnosed during a very particular phase in a woman's life: pregnancy. The incidence of cancer during pregnancy ranges from 0.07% to 0.1% of all cancer diagnoses, with an estimated increase of about 1 case per 1000 pregnancies. The most common malignant neoplasms during pregnancy include cervical cancer, breast cancer, melanoma, lymphomas, and leukemias [2]. Leukemias are relatively rare neoplasms, which correspond to less than 3.0% of all malignant neoplasms. Incidence of leukemia during pregnancy is small with the most frequent acute forms [2, 3].

A retrospective study from 2001 to 2011, which included 16 pregnant women with leukemia accompanied by prenatal care specialized in hemopathies and pregnancy at the University of São Paulo, diagnosed: acute lymphoid leukemia (ALL) in five cases (31.3%), acute myeloid leukemia (AML) in two cases (12.5%), and chronic myeloid leukemia (CML) in nine cases (56.3%). In cases of acute leukemias, two (28.6%) cases were diagnosed in the first trimester, two (28.6%) in

A. M. N. Machado (✉)
Stem Cell Transplantation Team of the Hospital Israelita Albert Einstein, São Paulo, Brazil

ABC Medical School, Santo André, Brazil
e-mail: andrea.novaes@einstein.br

P. M. R. de Souza
Stem Cell Transplantation Team of the Hospital Israelita Albert Einstein, São Paulo, Brazil

Oxford International Center for Palliative Care, Oxford, UK

Pain Committee for the Elderly of the Brazilian Society for the Study of Pain-SBED, São Paulo, Brazil

Bioethics Committee of Hospital Israelita Albert Einstein, São Paulo, Brazil

Oncology and Hematology Center of Hospital Israelita Albert Einstein, São Paulo, Brazil

© Springer Nature Switzerland AG 2021
C. W. P. Schmidt, K. M. Otoni (eds.), *Chemotherapy and Pharmacology for Leukemia in Pregnancy*, https://doi.org/10.1007/978-3-030-54058-6_11

the second, and three (42.9%) in the third. Two pregnant women with ALL diagnosed in the first trimester opted for therapeutic abortion. Four cases of acute leukemia received chemotherapy treatment during pregnancy, with a diagnosis established
after the 20th week. In a case of ALL with late diagnosis (30th week), chemotherapy was initiated after delivery. All pregnant women with acute leukemia developed
anemia and thrombocytopenia; four cases (57.1%) evolved with febrile neutropenia.
Of the pregnant women with CML, four used imatinib mesylate when they became
pregnant, three of them suspended in the first trimester, and one in the second.
During pregnancy, three (33.3%) did not require antineoplastic therapy after suspension of imatinib, and in six (66.7%) the following drugs were used: interferon
($n = 5$) and/or hydroxyurea ($n = 3$). In the group of pregnant women with CML,
anemia was found in four cases (44.4%) and plaquetopenia in one (11.1%).
Regarding perinatal results, in pregnancies complicated by acute leukemia, the
mean gestational age in childbirth was 32 weeks (standard deviation – SD = 4.4)
and the mean weight of the newborn was 1476 g (SD = 657 g). There were two
(40.0%) perinatal deaths (one fetal and one neonatal). In pregnancies complicated
by CML, the mean gestational age at delivery was 37.6 weeks (SD = 1.1) and the
mean weight of the newborn was 2870 g (SD = 516 g); there was no perinatal death
and no fetal abnormalities were detected. Therefore, high maternal and fetal morbidity was observed in pregnancies complicated by acute leukemia; while, in those
complicated by CML, maternal and fetal prognosis seems to be more favorable,
with greater ease in the management of complications [4].

During the trajectory of any oncological disease, patients and family members
may face an immense burden of suffering due to physical and emotional symptoms,
in addition to socioeconomic problems and spiritual issues generated by the disease
itself and/or its treatment, leading to severe impairment of quality of life [3–5].

During pregnancy, such suffering tends to be potentiated. All these dilemmas
related to difficult decisions involving the preservation of maternal life versus the
preservation of the integrity of the fetus are added, since when promoting alternative treatments with reduced risk of fetal impairment, one can significantly alter the
maternal prognosis [5]. And even if treatments of lower toxicity potential for the
fetus are considered, there are still risks of injury, which can be diverse, depending
on the drugs and dosages chosen.

It cannot be ignored that pregnancy is a unique phase in the life of woman with
intense bodily, emotional, and social changes. During this period, the pregnant
woman, her partner, and her family members develop several expectations regarding the expected child, which can be extremely shaken during the processing of
maternal illness, placing the pregnant woman at risk. In addition, there is a great
emotional impact of the risk of fetal damage when we talk about the treatment of a
maternal disease, generating feelings such as sadness, suffering at the prospect of
child loss, feeling of guilt for possible damage, and suffering caused to the child by
treatment, including the high risk of fetal death, in addition to the possibility of
death itself [5–7].

For the assessment and treatment of suffering resulting from physical, emotional,
economic and spiritual related to cancer illness, international organizations and

societies that play a leading role in combating cancer, such as WHO, the American Society of Clinical Oncology (ASCO), the European Society of Medical Oncology (ESMO), and the National Comprehensive Cancer Network (NCCN), recommend increasingly early integration of palliative care during the course of the disease. This recommendation results from the publication of an increasing number of randomized and controlled studies with a high level of evidence, which demonstrated the benefits of offering this type of care to cancer patients concomitant with the usual cancer treatment, determining improvement in mood, prognostic understanding, quality of life, and overall survival of the patient [8–10]. However, such studies do not include patients with hematological neoplasms, especially pregnant patients with solid or hematological neoplasms. Most studies correlating palliative care and pregnancy were constructed in the scenario of fetal illness and not maternal illness.

The first records of a care model using the concept of palliative care in pregnant women and fetal medicine date back to the 1990s, when there was the first medical discussion about the possibility of follow-up and planning of care for the fetus diagnosed with a lethal disease in the prenatal period, using family values as reference. This same team first proposed a follow-up model for families who decided to take term pregnancy after the diagnosis of lethal or high-mortality fetal malformations [6–8]. Since then, studies on perinatal palliative care have been growing. Even in the present day, there is an absolute lack of studies on appropriate palliative care models during pregnancy when it comes to maternal cancer illness.

Considered by the World Health Organization (WHO) as a priority in health and universal human law, palliative care represents an active and total response to problems arising from prolonged, progressive, and/or life-threatening diseases, based on an interdisciplinary approach whose primary objective is to provide the best possible quality of life to patients and their families [11]. It is a philosophy of health care that combines science and humanism in an attempt to prevent and treat suffering, aiming to care for all stages of a serious disease and should not be limited only to the final stage of life, as somebody still believes [12–14].

Acute leukemias have difficult management during pregnancy, and their treatment should be started quickly after diagnosis to reduce the risk of poor maternal prognosis, because without any treatment the disease is fatal. When the diagnosis occurs in the second and third trimesters of pregnancy, there is usually no need for interruption of pregnancy. However, when diagnosed in the first trimester, there is a higher risk of damage to the fetus. These points need to be widely discussed with patients and their peers to provide decision-making that addresses their values and preferences. In addition to maternal and fetal risks, issues related to possible repercussions for the woman's reproductive future must also be considered [15].

Thus, there is a need for involvement of a highly available, attentive interdisciplinary team that includes obstetricians, pediatricians, hematologists, psychologists, social workers, and palliative care specialists to manage all complex needs that may arise throughout treatment. Throughout the process, there will be numerous situations that demand the intervention of the palliative care team in conjunction with the primary care team, especially with regard to adequate control of symptoms related to disease and treatment, in addition to promoting discussions related to the values, desires, preferences, and decision-making of patients and their families.

According to the WHO, palliative care is defined as an "approach that improves the quality of life of patients and their families facing the problem associated with life-threatening illness, through the prevention and relief of suffering by means of early identificatio1n and impeccable assessment and treatment of pain and other problems, physical, psychosocial and spiritual" [12, 13].

Palliative care can be defined as the basic and fundamental principles that guide all actions and elect as a unit of care for the patient and his or her family, who must be cared for and respected in their principles, values, culture, and beliefs. These principles advocate the following [12, 13]:

1. It promotes relief from pain and other symptoms, using the best scientific evidence available; it ensures that patients have access to any measurement, drug or not, necessary for proper control of their symptoms, whether physical or not. Remember that in the scenario of pregnancy, it is essential that the use of medications be widely discussed with the obstetrician and pediatrician of the team in order to maintain adequate control of symptoms with the possible fetal risk suit. Consider planning all necessary measures to avoid drug withdrawal crisis in postpartum newborns when using medicines with this potential in the control of maternal symptoms.

2. It affirms life and sees death as a natural process. Patients should be assured of the means that enable them to live in the most active and productive way possible throughout the course of the disease, accompanying their modifications throughout the disease.

3. Do not rush or postpone death. Palliative care does not use measures that intentionally prolong life, in the sense that it does not employ artificial life-prolonging measures when they are not indicated. This does not mean restricting the necessary and appropriate investigations and treatments for each situation, and their rational use. There are bioethical discussions that may be appropriate in cases of need for prolongation of maternal life to enable fetal survival in extremely particular cases.

4. It integrates social, psychological, and spiritual aspects into care, according to the needs of patients, their families, and caregivers.

5. It promotes means that help the family deal with the disease and grief.

6. Preconize approach by multidisciplinary team.

7. It is applicable from the early stages of the disease, concomitantly with other therapies with curative intent.

8. It aims at improving quality of life and comfort, according to the expectation of patients and their families; it may even positively influence the course of the disease and survival.

9. It recommends effective communication with the family and the patient on diagnosis and prognosis, as well as the possibilities, risks, and benefits of possible treatments.

10. It ensures that the patient's decisions and preferences (or family members or legal representatives) are respected when the patient is unable to decide and there is no prior information about their preferences.

In 2016, the American Society of Oncology (ASCO) developed a project to offer high-quality palliative care for cancer patients [16]. These recommendations were reinforced in a new document published in 2018 [10]. It is not a publication that addresses specificities of the follow-up of pregnant women with cancer, but there is no reason for them to be excluded from these recommendations. The document has been divided into fundamental areas for good care and strongly recommends the following:

1. Early diagnosis and adequate management of symptoms: symptoms such as nausea, vomiting, diarrhea, dyspnea, and pain should be evaluated and administered. Patients with uncontrolled symptoms should be referred to specialized palliative care or other specialties, according to clinical indication.
2. Evaluation and psychosocial support since the beginning of the follow-up: the panel members agreed that there should be an initial psychosocial evaluation as well as an assessment of suffering. Anguish and suffering must be systematically evaluated.
3. Active approach to spiritual and cultural aspects: various elements of spiritual support were considered in order to provide a structure for the reception of expectations and hopes. Communication and language preferences should be evaluated and documented from a cultural perspective.
4. Enhanced communication for shared decisions: patients and families should be evaluated for preferences regarding how they want to receive information about cancer, prognosis, risks and benefits of treatment, treatment plan, and bad news; who participates in decision-making and to what extent. Oral and written documentation of the treatment plan should be provided to patients and the family with specific details about expectations of disease control, expected effects on symptoms and quality of life, expected duration and frequency of treatment, and justifications for the reassessment of the disease. Doubts and errors should be openly recognized and treated as soon as they are noticed.
5. Construction of an advanced care plan: discussion about the living will and end of life care should begin at the time of diagnosis of advanced cancer, with the assessment of patient and family availability in discussing early planning of care and any concerns that may arise.
6. Promotion of continuity of care with integration between the different levels of care: the panel members recorded the extreme need for coordination of care with primary care, high-complexity hospital, long-stay institutions, and hospice to promote continuous care according to the demands and progression of symptoms.
7. Provision of joint assistance by a team specialized in palliative care: routine gains must be carried out to determine the need for palliative care or for referral to specialized palliative care teams.

8. Support for those who care (formal, informal caregivers and health team): the panel participants agreed that physicians should approach the primary caregiver and include them in conversations about patient care. Caregivers attending clinical consultations with patients should be evaluated from a certain number of visits and those responsible should know how to contact physicians in emergency situations. Bereaved caregivers should receive support and have access to information about care resources if necessary. There must be constant open communication, respect, and care.
9. End-of-life care: the teams should have processes to assess symptoms, advise medication changes, and provide 24-hour support of the day, 7 days a week as the disease evolves. Identification of disease progression and finite symptoms should be accurate and rapid.

11.1 Final Considerations

Early integration of palliative care into cancer treatment has been increasingly recommended, since it can favor better care outcomes, including therapeutic planning, identification and adequate control of symptoms (physical, emotional, social, spiritual), sincere and effective communication, satisfaction with care, prevention of caregiver overload, and quality of life. For this care to occur, it is essential to involve a multidisciplinary and interdisciplinary team, bringing together knowledge, attitudes, and skills to help the patient adapt to life changes consequent to illness, promoting the necessary reflection to cope with this condition of threat to life not only to patients but also to their families. These are fundamental premises of palliative care advocated by WHO.

Despite the increasing understanding of the importance of palliative care, there are still important gaps among the most diverse populations of cancer patients. The scarcity of studies in the area in pregnant women with cancer diseases is a clear example and draws attention, since these are patients who, in addition to going through a very particular phase of life, may present with several difficulties related to the restricted use of drugs, which can compromise adequate symptomatic control. This post, it is perceived the need to carry out relevant studies that can better guide the practice in this scenario.

References

1. WHO. World cancer report 2014. Lyon; 2014 (ISBN 978-92-832-0443-5).
2. Pavlidis NA. Coexistence of pregnancy and malignancy. Oncologist. 2002;7(4):279–87.
3. Pejovic T, Schwartz PE. Leukemias. Clin Obstet Gynecol. 2002;45(3):866–78.
4. Nomura RMY, Igai AMK, Faciroli NC, Aguiar IN, Zugaib M. Maternal and perinatal results in pregnant women with leukemia. Rev Bras Ginecol Obstet. 2011;33(8):174–81.
5. Bolibio R, et al. Palliative care in fetal medicine. Rev Med (Sao Paulo). 2018;97(2):208–15.

6. Calhoun BC, Reitman JS, Hoeldtke NJ. Perinatal hospice: a response top artial birth abortion for infants with congenital defects. Issues Law Med. 1997;13(2):125–43.

7. Hoeldtke NJ, Calhoun BC. Perinatal hospice. Am J Obstet Gynecol. 2001;185(3):525–9. https://doi.org/10.1067/mob.2001.116093.

8. Bauman S, Temel ST. The integration of early palliative care with oncology care: the time has come for a new tradition. J Natl Compr Canc Netw. 2014;12(12):1763–71.

9. FERREL BR, et al. Integration of palliative care into standard oncology care: American Society of Clinical Practice Guidiline Update. J Clin Oncol. 2016;34:1–19.

10. OSMAN H, et al. Palliative care in the global setting: ASCO resource-stratified practice guideline. J Glob Oncol. 2018;4:1–24.

11. National Comprehensive Cancer Network. Palliative care (Version 2.2019). Available in: https://www.nccn.org/professionals/physician_gls/pdf/palliative.pdf. Access on 04/08/2019.

12. Connor S, Bermedo MC. Global atlas of palliative care at the end of life. Geneva/London: World Health Organization and Worldwide Palliative Care Alliance; 2014.

13. WHO, WHO. Palliative care. Available in: http://www.who.int/news-room/fact-sheets/detail/palliative-care. Access on 08/08/2019.

14. Twycross R. Palliative medicine: philosophy and ethical considerations. Bioethics. 2000;1(6):27–46.

15. Su WL, Liu JY, Kao WY. Management of pregnancy-associated acute leukemia. Eur J Gynaecol Oncol. 2003;24(3-4):251–4.

16. Bickel KE, et al. Defining high-quality palliative care in oncology practice: an American Society of Clinical Oncology/American Academy of Hospice and Palliative Medicine guidance statement. J Oncol Pract. 2016;12(9):828–38.

Index

© Springer Nature Switzerland AG 2021
C. W. P. Schmidt, K. M. Otoni (eds.), *Chemotherapy and Pharmacology
for Leukemia in Pregnancy*, https://doi.org/10.1007/978-3-030-54058-6

Printed in the United States
By Bookmasters